A GUIDE TO EXERCISE AND FITNESS EQUIPMENT

A GUIDE TO EXERCISE AND FITNESS EQUIPMENT

By the Editors of
Prevention® Magazine

Longmeadow Press

Notice

This book is intended as a reference volume only, not as a medical manual or guide to self-treatment. It is not intended as a substitute for the medical advice of physicians. The reader should regularly consult a physician in general, and particularly for any symptoms. If you suspect that you have a medical problem, we urge you to seek competent medical help. Keep in mind that exercise and nutritional needs vary from person to person, depending on age, sex, health status and individual variations. The information here is intended to help you make informative decisions about your health, not as a substitute for any treatment that may have been prescribed by your doctor.

A Guide to Exercise and Fitness Equipment

Copyright © 1987 Rodale Press, Inc. All Rights Reserved.

Cover Art © 1987 by Rodale Press

Library of Congress Cataloging-in-Publication Data

A guide to exercise and fitness equipment.

    (No-nonsense health guide)
    1. Exercise—Equipment and supplies. I. Prevention (Emmaus, Pa.) II. Series.
[DNLM: 1. Equipment and Supplies—popular works. 2. Exertion—popular works. 3. Physical Fitness—popular works. QT 260 C758]
GV543.C368   1987   613.7′028   87-2687
ISBN 0-681-40132-X   paperback

Special thanks to Catherine Cassidy for compiling and editing the information in this book.

Book design by Acey Lee and Lisa Gatti

Photographs by Kevin Bubbenmoyer: pp. 25, 58, bottom; Angelo Caggiano: p. 43; Carl Doney: p. 7; Donna Hornberger: pp. 9, bottom, 71; Mark Lenny: pp. 3, 4, 5; Mitchell T. Mandel: pp. 45, 46, 51, 52, 58, top; Alison Miksch: p. 28; Pat Seip: pp. 50, 57; Christie C. Tito: pp. 9, top, 19, 22, 24, 33, 59, 67, 68, 85, 86; Sally Shenk Ullman: pp. 64, 65, 66, 69, 76, 77; Rodale Press Photography Department: pp. 36, 38; photo courtesy of *Runner's World:* p. 42.

2   4   6   8   10   9   7   5   3   1   paperback

Contents

Getting Fit Faster and Easier

Not so long ago, people who wanted to get into shape had few options. They could don sweats and cruise along streets, highways and parks—whether they *liked* to run or not. Or they could join a body-building gym and mingle with Arnold Schwarzenegger look-alikes to the sound of heavy barbells clanging—and *try* not to feel self-conscious.

Today, people know they can get the same benefits from cycling, rowing or swimming that they can from running. And a smorgasbord of weight machines is available to help people build strength in the comfort of their own home—or a friendly neighborhood "family" fitness center. With this interest in varied activity come dozens—no, *hundreds*—of different kinds of exercise and fitness equipment. And the right equipment can, in fact, help you to get fit faster and easier.

Perhaps you've heard that rowing is great because it exercises the large muscles of your arms, legs, back and upper body yet doesn't stress your joints the way running does. A rowing machine, which imitates the motions of rowing on water, is the perfect solution.

Suppose swimming is your game but you know that swimming

endless laps does only so much. You want to swim faster or harder—or just add some kick to your routine. Enter swim fins, webbed mitts, kickboards and other paraphernalia—equipment that's not only fun to use but also improves your technique.

You say that bicycling appeals to you, but all too often you skip your scheduled jaunts due to dark of night, heavy downpours or noisy traffic? You'll find yourself working out more regularly—and getting fit right on schedule—if you heft your bike onto a wind-load trainer, a stand designed to accommodate your bike when you'd rather stay put while you ride. Or you can buy a stationary bike and cycle in the privacy and comfort of your own home—even while you watch TV or read—without getting bored or discouraged.

And so it goes. For every mode of exercise, it seems there are many gadgets or gizmos to enhance your workout, including indoor ski simulators, minitrampolines, weighted jump ropes, wrist and ankle weights. There are even lightweight monitors that, when strapped to your wrist or torso, measure your pulse or give you other information to take the guesswork out of gauging your performance.

Faced with so many choices, how does a consumer decide what, if any, fitness equipment to use or buy? Are all stationary bikes basically alike, or do you, in fact, "get what you pay for"? Which is more economical, working out in a gym or buying a set of weight machines to use at home? Do items such as sauna belts and vibrating machines really melt away flab the way the ads say they do?

To help you decide how to best spend your fitness dollars, we've reviewed a representative sampling of exercise and fitness equipment, ranging from a simple, inexpensive jump rope to the ultimate product of computer technology and exercise science—a fully computerized exercise machine with a price tag of $16,500. Most equipment, however, is somwehere in between. The trick is to learn what features to look for *before* you buy, to make sure the equipment suits your needs.

Even if you already own some sort of workout equipment, we hope you'll consult this book when considering additions to your collection or when replacing items that no longer meet your needs. As with any consumer merchandise, the prices quoted and the equipment described may have changed since we printed this information. Please contact the manufacturers or your local dealer for current prices and other purchasing information.

A Bike for All Seasons

Okay, it's October. After a sweet summer of virtuous fitness—jumping into the pool each evening after work, running on the weekends—it's getting colder and you're running out of exercise steam. Winters and bad weather don't have to mean curtains for your workouts—not when stationary bikes are ready, willing and able to provide you with a great indoor workout that will quickly guarantee you all the guilt-free evenings you want.

"Stationary bicycling can be an excellent indoor activity," say Bryant Stamford, Ph.D., and Arthur Weltman, Ph.D., two physical fitness experts who write a sportsmedicine advice column in *The Physician and Sportsmedicine.* "It involves the large leg muscles; most people can cycle for at least 30 minutes; and if the resistance on the cycle can be adjusted, it is possible to sufficiently elevate the heart rate."

What to Look For in an Exercise Bike

According to *Bicycling* magazine and *Consumer Reports,* both of which tested various exercise bikes on the market, there are basics you should look for when you head out to shop for a stationary bike.

- An easy-to-use resistance device. Since adjusting the resistance is the way you'll reach your target heart rate, this is a must on your bike—and it should also be within easy reach.
- A smooth ride. The bikes that give you this have sturdy frames that don't wiggle or flex. Check it out with a test ride.
- Adjustable handlebars and seat. Since other members of your family might use the bike, you'll want to be certain these adjustments can be made easily.
- Distance and speed devices. These will also help you stay within your target heart rate. A speedometer (miles per hour) or tachometer (revolutions per minute) helps you stay at an even speed. A timer or an odometer (distance) can help you calculate how long or far you've cycled.
- Comfortable pedals and seat. You're going to be on it all winter, so you'd better be sure it's suited to your feet and posterior. Some bikes come with pedal straps that help keep your feet from slipping off. However, you can also buy straps at a bike shop.

Four Outstanding Bikes

Here are four bikes recommended by the experts at *Bicycling* magazine.

The Tunturi Professional.   Known best for its massive, 51-pound flywheel, the Tunturi Professional is about as rugged and smooth riding as a stationary bike can be. For someone serious about getting a workout, welcome features include a friction-control device (a stem-mounted lever with numbered stops) and adjustable handlebars that swivel forward, back, up and down. "Straight down, the rider finds himself in a familiar roadbike crouch; straight up, the bike fits more like the old, venerable three-speed," according to *Bicycling*'s testers. Instrumentation is adequate but not state of the art (a 60-minute timer plus a pedaling cadence gauge). More detailed fitness feedback is available, however, by comparing cadence and tension settings with a chart provided in the owner's manual. The bike could use toe clips and a

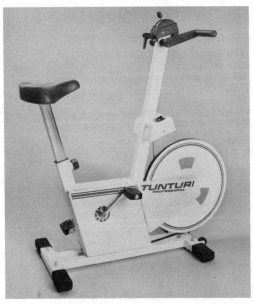

Tunturi Professional

slightly more adjustable seat, but other than those minor drawbacks, the Tunturi's reputation as the Rolls Royce of stationary bikes seems reasonably well deserved.

The Monark Mark II.   The Monark II is designed to feel like an honest-to-goodness racing bike. It's got drop-style handlebars, a narrow saddle, standard-length pedals, toe clips and straps. What it also has, however, is a surprising amount of stability. Despite having a lighter flywheel and greater portability than the Tunturi, the Monark II holds up well under hard pedaling. Instrumentation is good (you get readouts on revolutions per minute, speed and workload in watts), and seat adjustment, unlike with the Tunturi, provides all the fore-and-aft possibilities of a standard bike. All in all a very good unit, especially suited to avid racing and touring cyclists.

The Schwinn Bio-Dyne.   The strength of the Schwinn Bio-Dyne is its ability to monitor a pedaler's efforts. By maintaining a cadence of 70, 75 or 90 revolutions per minute and then reading a load-indicator dial, a rider can get a precise picture (in terms of kilopond meters per minute) of how hard he's working. *Bicycling*'s testers were impressed with the "silky-smooth ride" of the Bio-Dyne, and they liked

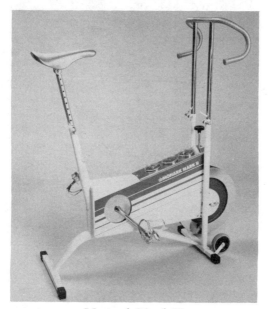

Monark Mark II

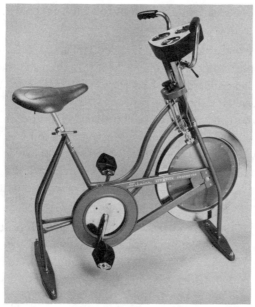

Schwinn Bio-Dyne

its overall sturdiness. What they did not relish, however, was the unit's fixed-gear chain drive, an arrangement that means the pedals keep turning for several seconds after the rider has stopped. The design achieves exceptional smoothness but at the expense of safety. Overall, however, the Bio-Dyne impressed *Bicycling* as being a very worthwhile bike.

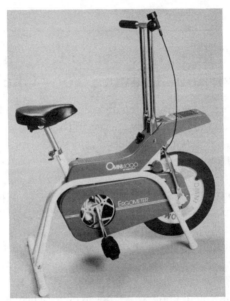

Omni 4000

The Omni 4000. "A shining example of a moderately priced, well-made bicycle that could be top drawer with just a few modifications," said *Bicycling* of the Omni. What bothered testers most was the bike's resistance device, which tended to grab and slip, resulting in unstable readings coming through the workload indicator. All kinds of good fitness information comes in the Omni's training manual, however. "The crash course on human ergometry dives right into the technical side of fitness. An engineer's delight," reported the testers. Delightful, too, they said, were the Omni's counterweighted pedals (designed to remain upright for easy entry), fully adjustable seat and conveniently located resistance-control knob.

Wind-Load Trainers:
Spinning with the Wind

Another way to cycle indoors is with a wind-load trainer, a bicyclelike contraption that provides the pedaling resistance of a road bike. Wind-load trainers have come a long way since they entered the marketplace about eight years ago. Some early models were loud, complicated to set

The Port-a-Cycle: Cycling
without Leaving Your Chair

You've tried eight million different times of the day to exercise—and something always gets in the way.

You hate exercising outside in cold weather.

You'd join a health club, but there isn't a decent or convenient one in your area.

If you fit any of the above descriptions (or any others that prevent you from getting the exercise you want), the Port-a-Cycle might be just the gadget you need.

Looking strangely like half an exercise bike, the Port-a-Cycle is, in fact, just that! It has all the features you're likely to see on a regular exercise bike, including pedals, a timer and a tension-adjustment knob. But it doesn't have a bike seat or handlebars.

To use it, you attach its straps to the rungs on your chair and start pedaling from your seat. Because of its size, it's easier to hide in a corner of your office than a full-size exercise bike (and it may be easier to explain to the higher-ups, too). It's also fairly portable (it weighs 25 pounds and the manufacturer sells a tote bag that you can transport it in), so you can take it on vacations or even business trips.

Finally, it makes it easy to do two things at once, like pedaling while you catch up on all that business reading and correspondence.

up, and tended to bounce across the floor when you got off the saddle to really honk on the pedals. Still, those trainers cost *less* than a regular stationary bike. Even though the fans made noise, they provided resistance to your pedaling that came close to the feel of the road. Best of all, the trainer enabled you to "cycle" for an hour a day during the cold, wet, winter doldrums.

Today's wind trainers are quieter, more stable and durable and less

The Port-a-Cycle costs $326 and is available from sporting goods dealers. An optional carrying bag costs $38. If you can't locate a retailer in your area who carries the bike, contact Jayfro Corporation, 976 Hartford Turnpike, P.O. Box 400, Waterford, CT 06385 (800-243-0533).

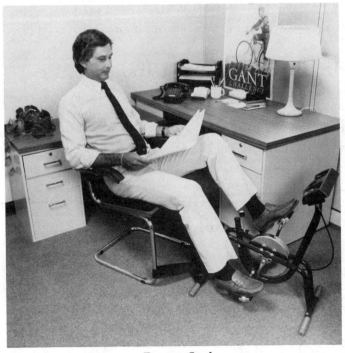

Port-a-Cycle

expensive. Best of all, most are very easy to set up. If a beautiful winter day beckons you outdoors, you can quickly pop the bike off the stand and head out into the real world.

Typically, the stand for each of these trainers is metal tubing shaped into an "I." The "I" rests on the floor, and two upright supports branch off—one to support the bike by the front fork and the other to support it under the bottom bracket. At the back of the trainer, where the rear wheel will be, two fans attach to either end of a roller assembly. As the rear wheel turns the roller, the roller spins the fans, which provide pedaling resistance. Hence the name, "wind-load trainer."

Most wind-load trainers require you to set up your bike in roughly the same way. You remove the bike's front wheel, rest the front fork and bottom bracket on the upright supports, secure the bike, and off you go!

The major difference among trainers lies in how the bike is fitted and attached to each one. If you have only one bike, you'll want it to be fairly accessible for riding outdoors—it should come on and off that trainer without much work. If you have two bikes and one can stay on the trainer most of the time, ease of assembly won't be your top priority.

Selecting a Good Wind Trainer

When you choose a wind trainer, you want the union between it and your bike to be a long, healthy one. If you're concerned about not marring your bike's gleaming paint job, examine the bottom bracket support where trainer and bike intersect. Most of the trainers have

---

Read while You Ride

As great as they are for the body, stationary bikes can get a little boring for the brain. J. Oglaend, Inc., to the rescue. The company manufactures a stationary-bike reading stand. So if you're just not the "Today Show" type, give Oglaend a call at (800) 828-1186, or drop them a line at 40 Radio Circle, Mt. Kisco, NY 10549-0096, to see what they've got.

either plastic or rubber-padded supports to protect the bike from scratches. Some units come with an additional rubber cover for extra protection.

The fans are both the most important and the most stressed parts

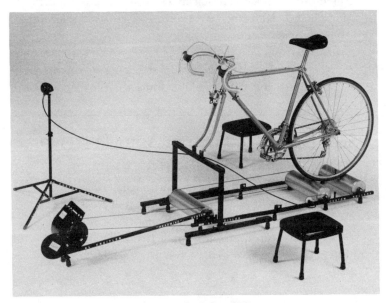

Kreitler Wind-Load System

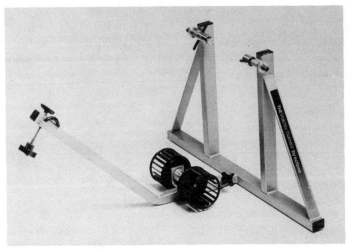

Eclipse Vortex Wind Trainer (requires no wheel removal)

of wind-load trainers. Fans also are susceptible to damage in transit; the somewhat delicate blades may be bent if the unit is banged around. In any case, they are easily replaced. Wind trainers should have rust-resistant finishes—sweat can quickly corrode a nonresistant finish. Good finishes include chrome/epoxy, polyurethane, baked resin/brushed chrome or chrome rubber.

When you're out on the road, riding fast creates a natural cooling breeze. When you're working out indoors and not going anywhere, the heat—and sweat—can build up. Some manufacturers offer optional air

Seat Covers to Pamper Your Posterior

If you've ever spent Monday walking around like John Wayne because of sore haunches you acquired during a long stint on your exercise bike, the new, supersoft, bicycle seat covers may be the answer to your problem.

We put six seat covers through the rigors of testing. The results of the tests appear in the accompanying table.

Manufacturer	Suggested Retail Price (1984)	Comfort Score (1 to 10)
Allyn Air Seat Allyn Air Seat Co. 18 Millstream Rd. Woodstock, NY 12498 (914) 679-2051	$10.00	9.1
Cannondale Sheepskin Cannondale Corp. 9 Brookside Pl. Georgetown, CT 06829 (203) 544-9430	$10.95	8.7

diversion systems to channel the breeze from the rotating fans to your body. Metal shrouds cover the fans to direct a cooling breeze to your working muscles. The most effective designs connect tubing to the shrouds to better direct the air flow.

When riding a trainer, you want to be able to concentrate on training. If the apparatus is wobbling and threatening to throw you into the television, revolutions per minute are the last thing you think about. That's the advantage of built-in stability—with the trainer you feel safe and can lose yourself in your favorite fitness fantasy.

Manufacturer	Suggested Retail Price (1984)	Comfort Score (1 to 10)
Grab On Coveralls Grab On Products 100 N. Avery Walla Walla, WA 99362 (509) 529-9800	$9.95	9.3
Hydroseat (Racing) **Leather Cover** International Aqua Products 1306 7th St., NW Rochester, MN 55901 (507) 288-4847	$24.95	10.0
Hydroseat (Women's) **Vinyl Cover** International Aqua Products 1306 7th St., NW Rochester, MN 55901 (507) 288-4847	$17.95	9.1
Spenco Saddle Pad Spenco Medical Corp. P.O. Box 2501 Waco, TX 76702 (800) 433-3334	$24.95	10.0

One If by Land: Rowing Machines

When you think of rowing, what image immediately comes to mind? Slaves in galleys propelling ancient vessels of war? Viking explorers? English gentlemen competing at Henley-on-Thames on lovely summer afternoons? Ivy League college crew teams?

Rowing is all that and more.

Rowing is, in fact, one of the most versatile and accessible aerobic sports. We're talking about rowing as a sport—for competition or exercise—not meandering around in a rowboat. Its pluses are numerous.

- Rowing is a great aerobic exercise for people with orthopedic problems because it doesn't place a great deal of stress on joints.
- It exercises most of the large muscle groups of the body.
- You can do it in your home or office with the help of a rowing machine, which simulates the water's resistance with tension devices.

Since most people don't have ready access to open water, the most widely used equipment for rowing is found in the gym and the home. Rowing machines are designed to allow you to imitate the arm, leg, back and upper body action of actual rowing. And you get the same aerobic benefits available from rowing on the water.

The better machines have a moving seat that slides when you pull and push the oars and a means of adjusting the resistance so that you can increase the intensity of the exercise. Some have an ergometer for measuring speed and the distance you've rowed.

No matter where you choose to do your rowing, you can count on a pretty good caloric output. Vigorous rowing can use up about 600 calories an hour, and an easy row can expend about half of that.

Choosing the Right Rower

Before you rush out to buy a rowing machine, keep in mind the following recommendations:

- Look for smooth seat action. Rowers have sliding seats so that your legs get into the exercise act. A jittery ride won't be pleasant, especially after you've been at it for 20 minutes or so.
- Make sure the seat is comfortable and well padded. You're going to be spending a lot of time perched on it.
- The seat should be able to slide a good distance—enough so that you can fully extend your legs.
- The frame should be solid enough so that the machine doesn't jump around the floor every time you stroke.
- The footpads should be adjustable to an angle that's comfortable for you and have a bar or Velcro strap to keep your feet in place.
- Make sure the rowing arms are made of sturdy tubing—you don't want them to bend under the force of your stroke.
- Look for adjustable resistance, so that you can continue to make your workouts more difficult as you become more fit.

Bob Goldman, D.O., chairman of the Amateur Athletic Union's Sports Medicine Committee and director of sportsmedicine research at Chicago College of Osteopathic Medicine, is independently evaluating all types of exercise equipment in a project called the High Tech Equipment Research Study. Although he concedes that he has not evaluated all of the estimated 200 rowing machines on the market, he has put a fair number through their paces.

The machines he recommends are listed here. "Of the rowers I've analyzed, these are the ones that are produced by good companies, with good research and design departments and service," says Dr. Goldman. "Knock-offs of the top rowing machines, of which there are plenty, are often made of inferior materials that won't hold up."

The Tunturi TRM.   These Finnish-made machines are imported by Amerec. The TRM was the first rowing machine to provide resistance using hydraulic cylinders (like shock absorbers). It costs about $200. The TRM 2 is more high tech than the TRM, with sealed ball-bearing rollers for a smoother ride. "These are durable rowers and good for people looking in the lower price range," says Dr. Goldman. Cost: $275. Contact Amerec Corporation, P.O. Box 3825, Bellevue, WA 98009 (800-426-0858).

The West Bend 5100 and 5200.   These are also durable, well-made machines in the lower price range, says Dr. Goldman. The 5100 features dual hydraulic cylinders that provide resistance for the rowing arms and pivoting foot pedals that are also adjustable. Cost: $279.95. The 5200 has a slightly longer rail designed for extra-tall people, to allow full leg extension. It also features a stroke counter and a timer/stopwatch. Cost: $349.95. Contact West Bend Company, West Bend, WI 53095 (414-334-6909).

Precor rowing machines.   Precor is an innovative company that makes some of the most well thought-out exercise equipment on the market, says Dr. Goldman. "They use lighter materials and intelligent construction to come up with very strong machines." There are two lines of rowers. The newer M series features a rower that is totally silent, says Dr. Goldman. Cost: $365 to $600. The company's other rowers, numbered 600, 612, 615e, 620, 620e and 630e, range in size, features and price, from $185 to $600. Contact Precor, P.O. Box 1018, Redmond, WA 98052 (800-662-0606).

The Hydra-Fitness Pro-Row 2000.   "This is a powerfully built machine that will last forever," says Dr. Goldman. It inclines slightly up at the rear of the machine for a tougher workout and an easier glide back to the starting position. The Pro-Row 2000 costs $995 and can be converted into a strength-training machine that will allow you to do chest presses and abdominal exercises. There's also a Pro-Row 1000 for $895, which is just a rower without the other

Building Endurance

Begin your rowing program by mixing rowing (12 to 20 strokes per minute) with walking. From Week 2 through Week 12, mix brisk rowing (20 strokes per minute) with recovery rowing of 12 strokes per minute. Complete each routine three to four times weekly, with a rest day between workouts.

Week	Rowing (min.)	Recovery (min.)	Rowing (min.)	Recovery (min.)	Number of Times	Total (min.)
1	3	2	0	0	6	30
2	3	2	0	0	6	30
3	4	1	0	0	6	30
4	4	1	3	2	3	30
5	4	1	0	0	6	30
6	4	1	5	1	3	30
7	9	1	0	0	3	30
8	13	2	0	0	2	30
9	14	1	0	0	2	30
10	20	1	9	0	1	30
11	25	1	4	0	1	30
12	30	0	0	0	1	30

features. Contact Hydra-Fitness, P.O. Box 599, 2121 Industrial Boulevard, Belton, TX 76513 (800-433-3111; in Texas: 800-792-3013).

The Universal ComputeRow.   This is a completely electronic device that will last under any traffic, says Dr. Goldman. It is fully computerized and can be adjusted for time, distance, stroke resistance and cadence and for racing against an imaginary opponent. It also lets you know the amount of work you've done and how many calories you've burned. You can adjust it for two different workouts, an aerobic one and a strength-conditioning one. The strength workout is three times harder. Cost: $1,855. Contact Universal Fitness Products, P.O. Box 1270, Cedar Rapids, IA 52406 (800-553-7901).

Training Tools for Water Workouts

Fish, ducks and smart swimmers all have something in common: They help themselves swim faster by using fins, webbed feet or a variation of these. But only swimmers can *choose* their swimming aids. And we can choose today from a growing pool of equipment, including fins, webbed mitts, paddles, kickboards and more.

Many people are intimidated by these training tools, though. They think that only racers need them or can use them. They're wrong. Anyone who wants to be a better swimmer needs them. Masters swim clubs, whose members are primarily recreational swimmers who are 25 or older, regularly incorporate kicking and pulling drills into their workouts, as do high school and college teams.

Why? Because these swimmers want more than just exercise. They want improvement. And you don't improve your swimming by doing endless laps. You improve your swimming by improving your technique. For that, you need tools that are designed to isolate specific stroke components and enhance your efficiency in the water.

The right training tools can also make good work of stationary "water exercises" and stretches. Especially if you are injured or over-

weight, water workouts can offer superb exercise without the jarring
and pounding of other activities. (See your local sporting goods dealer
for the types of items we discuss here.)

Strong-Arm It

Because so much of your swimming speed depends on your arms,
begin your training there.

Paddles.   Traditional rigid plastic hand paddles increase the
load on the shoulders and arms and help you develop a much-desired
"feel for the water." This in turn enables you to get better traction.
When used in moderation, paddles will quickly improve arm strength.

Hand fins.   A new product called The Web is a flexible nylon
glove that comes close to making humans amphibious. These hand fins
cause you to catch gallons of water and increase strength. Plus, because
they are flexible, they make you acutely aware of even the slightest
stroke imbalance.

Wrist and ankle floats.   One way to add to the resistance of
the water and get even more out of a stationary water workout is to wear
floats (inflatable cuffs) on your wrists or ankles as you exercise. Since
the water pushes up on these light, air-filled swim aids, you'll have to
exert extra energy as you force your arms or legs down under the water.

Leg floats.   Pull-buoys are leg floats constructed of two foam
cylinders attached by an adjustable strap. They're commonly used with
paddles to further isolate upper body motion. You place them between
your legs at thigh level to keep your lower body afloat while your upper
body toils on.

Fin-ishing Touches

After you wipe out your arms, you can put on some fins and work
your leg muscles.

Foot fins.   Although sprinters need a strong kick, middle- and
long-distance swimmers should kick for stability rather than propul-
sion. Either way, you should use fins to develop leg strength and ankle

flexibility. Stiffer and larger blades will make you work harder, and you will notice that the difference in your stroke speed while wearing fins will carry over to your no-fin sessions.

Foam kickboards.   To completely isolate your kick, grab a foam kickboard and push off from the wall. The board keeps you afloat while you concentrate on kicking from the hip and producing little or no splash.

Stationary Swimming

Swimming in place builds strength while avoiding the need for a clear shot at an open lane in a crowded pool.

Tethers.   Made of rubber tubing that can be attached to poolside, tethers will allow you to swim nowhere fast. It's like swimming while

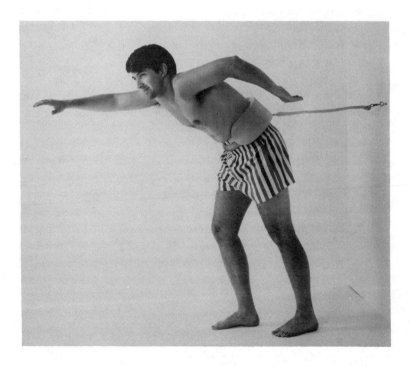

Swimmercizer

towing a barge full of people (a la Jack LaLanne pulling people around Alcatraz), but if you have a tiny pool, this may be the solution. The Lifeline Swim Trainer and the Swimmercizer are tethers for both the pool and the weight room. When you're not using the tether in the water, it performs well as a resistance device to develop strength.

Suit Yourself

Other accessories that may make water training more effective are drag suits, which catch extra water and slow your progress (that's why competitive swimmers wear two or three suits when training).

For cold-water swims, be sure to wear a neoprene wet suit and cap. Body Glove and O'Neill make all styles, from short vests to full suits, some of which have different thicknesses for arms and shoulders. Many swimsuit makers have added neoprene caps to their line in response to the boom in triathlon and open-water swims.

Earplugs and noseclips may make you more comfortable in the water. And for extra information about style, there are mirrors like the Swimsee, which may be placed on the bottom of the pool to help you see what you're doing wrong.

If you are afraid of open water, try the swim cabinet from AquaMotion. For a mere $4,000, it allows you to remove yourself from the world and effectively drown your sorrows. Just remember to emerge for feedings and showers.

Getting Your Ski Legs

One of the major frustrations of cross-country skiing is that lack of access to snow prevents you from performing your sport. Unless you live near a ski resort or in the very snowy North, there are likely to be long stretches of winter when the closest you come to the fluffy stuff is during your annual viewing of *White Christmas.*

But with the help of devices like roller skis and indoor cross-country ski exercisers, you can ski your heart out no matter what the weather.

Outdoor Cross-Country Skiing— Without the Snow

Roller skis are neat little pieces of equipment that allow you to train the Nordic way on dry ground. They are two normal-looking skis that are attached to wheels and roll along the road like roller skates.

You can use your own poles and boots with roller skis, but you have to get new bindings to attach to the skis themselves.

We asked several cross-country skiers to try out one brand of roller skis called SwedSki. They all thought the skis provided a good simulation of cross-country skiing and would be an excellent way to prepare for and stay in shape for the ski season.

"They'd be very good for practicing technique, because it's actually harder than skiing on snow," said one tester. "When you snow ski, there's a track in the snow to help you keep your balance. With roller skis, you must rely on your own balancing technique."

Because the wheels on the skis are rounded on all sides, it is possible to perform typical cross-country ski moves like the snowplow. The rear wheel also locks when you push off, so you can't slip backward.

The testers thought you'd be limited as to where you could work out with SwedSki. "You must have a well-paved surface, such as a parking lot or a newly paved street," said one. The other suggested

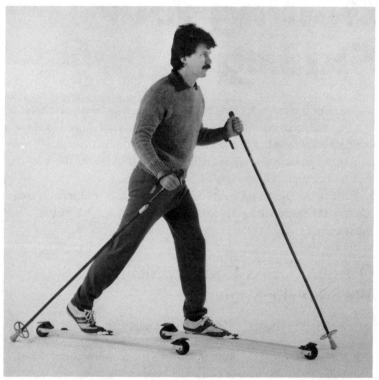

SwedSki

wearing knee and elbow pads, in case you fall onto a hard street. Because street surfaces are rougher than snow, one tester suggested covering the tips of your regular ski poles with the kinds of rubber stoppers used on the ends of canes.

The manufacturers of SwedSki tout their skis as an alternative to jogging. So we asked a runner who doesn't ski to try them out as well. He and our experienced cross-country ski testers agreed: You'd have a pretty difficult time learning to use the roller skis if you didn't have some experience with real skis before you started.

"I felt so awkward," said the runner. "It was like the first time I went roller skating—except this time I had skis to deal with as well!"

SwedSki is available at sporting goods and ski stores or directly from the manufacturer. The roller skis cost about $179. To order them directly, contact Continental Trading Corporation, 6600 France Avenue South, Minneapolis, MN 55435 (612-920-0108).

Nordic Trainers: The Inside Track

You can cycle, row or run in the privacy of your home—but did you know you can also cross-country ski indoors?

The NordicTrack cross-country ski exerciser consists of an oak frame in which a flywheel has been placed. The motion of your legs (on the cross-country skis attached) moves the flywheel and simulates the action of skis over snow. Your hands grip cords that you pull to simulate the poling motion of the cross-country skier.

Sound complicated? It really isn't, once you've learned the basic arm/leg coordination. In fact, increased coordination and balance are two of the benefits to be gained by exercising this way. So even if you're a klutz starting out, you will improve, according to NordicTrack users we contacted.

To learn more about this novel form of indoor exercise, we asked a group of exercisers who use the machine regularly to demonstrate it. We also contacted another NordicTrack user, the Institute of Health, Exercise and Athletic Rehabilitation (HEAR) in Red Bank, New Jersey.

As a preparation for cross-country skiing, our users ranked it high. They said that the NordicTrack can simulate a hard, outdoor workout.

Said one cross-country skier who used the machine to prepare for the season: "It also cut down on the soreness I usually feel after the first day out, especially in the muscles along my upper back and arms."

But NordicTrack has other fitness benefits, whether you ski or not. It gives you a harder workout than other, sit-down exercise machines, because you must support your whole body, according to HEAR physical therapist Pat Dunphy. It also works more muscle groups, especially in the buttocks area.

The NordicTrack can also be used as a rehabilitation tool, says Dunphy. Compared to other forms of exercise, HEAR finds it excellent for neck and back pain sufferers. "Instead of your heels hitting the ground, you use a sliding motion. That means there's less shock and pounding on joints and muscles," she says. "Because you're standing, there's less strain on the structures of the lower back, too."

Runners who are recovering from injuries but want to stay fit also use the NordicTrack at HEAR. Dunphy says it's especially good for runners with knee problems who might aggravate their condition using an exercise bike.

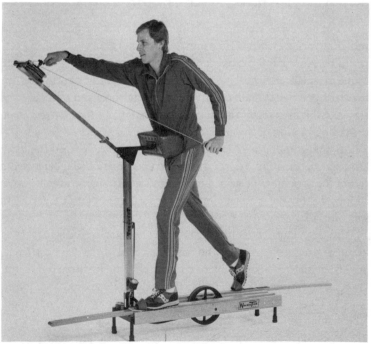

NordicTrack

For Downhill Racers

What can you do to prepare your legs for the demands of downhill skiing? Riding a bike, running, lifting weights or jumping rope are what the experts have always recommended— until Ski Legs appeared, that is. The device, which consists of a pair of partial skis that are strapped to your boots, is designed to allow skiers to simulate the action of skiing at home.

And our testers found that Ski Legs really does work. Moments after it arrived in our office, we had assembled it, donned our shiny new boots, grabbed our graphite poles, and "hit the slopes." After a few minutes of schussing in the hallway, our quads and calves began shouting that it was time for a hot-chocolate break.

The Ski Legs unit is fully adjustable, enabling the user to work on perfecting balancing skills and achieving a tight parallel form. Its well-illustrated instruction book is full of helpful tips on technique. The suggested retail price of Ski Legs is $200. You may find Ski Legs in your local ski shop, where it's used for boot-fitting, or contact Questek Corporation, 19201 Parthenia Street, Northridge, CA 91324.

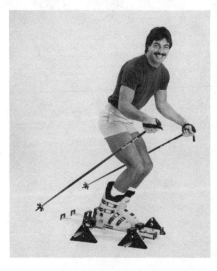

Ski Legs

One of the biggest criticisms we heard from people who hadn't used the NordicTrack before was that they felt so clumsy starting out. "It's like learning how to ride a two-wheeled bike for the first time!" said one frustrated beginner.

But regular users said the motion isn't difficult once you get the hang of it. Ed Pauls, the mechanical engineer who designed NordicTrack, recommends learning the arm motion first. Then balance your lower body against the cushion provided and use a light jogging stride to learn the leg motion. When you combine the two motions, use a quick, rhythmic stride and *don't* think too hard about what you're doing. Just relax and think about something else. The NordicTrack, which comes with instructions and a training program, costs around $470 for the at-home version. For more information, contact PSI, 124 Columbia Court, Chaska, MN 55318 (800-328-5888).

Fitness by Leaps and Bounds

Jumping for exercise—sounds like child's play, doesn't it? With rebounders and jump ropes selling like hotcakes and visible in gyms across the country these days, though, it's plain that leaping and bounding is here to stay. But is it viable aerobic exercise? And if so, what kind of equipment makes jumping and bounding a good exercise bet?

Rebounders: Fun, but Are They Aerobic?

Rebounders (or minitrampolines, as they're also called) are everywhere these days. Because you can run, leap or practice any number of go-for-broke exercises on them, their advocates say they are loads of fun and much less boring than other forms of indoor exercise.

And some experts believe they're safer, too. That's because rebounders absorb most of the shock of landing so there's less stress on joints. You might be less vulnerable to injury than you would be with more stressful exercises like running.

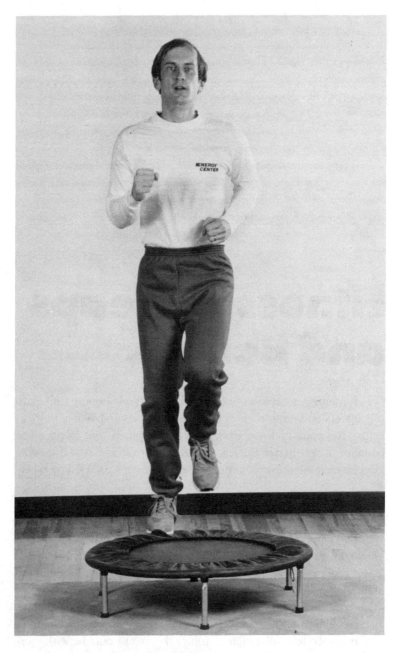

Rebounder (minitrampoline)

But will rebounders increase your aerobic endurance—one of the key measures of fitness? Early research had suggested they would. But more recent studies indicate that it is extremely difficult to keep your heart rate high enough to achieve much in the way of lasting aerobic endurance, according to Bryant Stamford, Ph.D., director of the Exercise Physiology Laboratory at the University of Louisville, Kentucky.

"Yes, if you're extremely dedicated and willing to really kick and move around a lot, you can get your heart rate up," Dr. Stamford says. "But the chances of getting someone to maintain that kind of choreography for 30 minutes a day are questionable."

Dr. Stamford says the other, more rhythmic exercises, like running and cycling, require less mental concentration and may be easier to maintain. "Rebounding may be more enjoyable, but the question you have to ask yourself is, 'Am I getting an aerobic workout?' "

Beginning exercisers will probably be initially successful in getting their heart rate up, "but a regular jogger would probably be disappointed," he says.

Dr. Stamford's views were confirmed by a study done at the University of Minnesota in Minneapolis. The findings were presented at a meeting of the American College of Sports Medicine. The researchers asked 20 sedentary women to bounce and run in place on minitramps for two 15-minute sessions (with a 5-minute rest between them) for 12 weeks. At the end of the study, the women had only "minimal improvement" in cardiovascular fitness. The researchers could find no change in the group's average weight, percentage of body fat or cholesterol levels.

We tried two firmer versions of the original trampoline-type rebounder, the Rebound Jogging Board and the Jogging Square. Both have solved a number of problems, but neither could be said to be what the doctor ordered for effective aerobic exercise.

"Combines a firm jogging surface with the resiliency of a springboard, enabling the body to get a firm yet cushioned workout," says the Gerstung Company of its Rebound Jogging Board. What they do not tell you, however, is that staying at the peak of the Jogging Board's crowned configuration is no easy task. "It takes more concentration than someone who's used to running is going to want to invest," said one marathoner we put aboard the unit. "The amount of spring provided is interesting, though. If it were bigger, I might have been able to get into it."

For rope skippers, the Jogging Board's 18- by 24-inch usable area was a frustration, also, as was its bowed shape. A nice idea, the Jogging Board. And well constructed. But other than providing an occasional fling, it's unlikely the $99 unit would keep as much company with your feet as with your closet.

And even less likely to win your heart would be the Jogging Board's even smaller little brother—the $70 Jogging Square. While the Jogging Board gets its bounce from its curved configuration, the Jogging Square relies on its "heavy-duty foam legs." Maybe too heavy.

"It didn't feel very different from jogging on just a carpet," said one tester. "And unless I had the unit on a carpet, it tended to move around under heavy use. I don't think I'd use it."

So if you're going to use a minitramp, use it in conjunction with other aerobic exercises. Or get up there and really jump your heart out. And don't forget to monitor your pulse to be certain you're reaching your target rate.

Jump for Fitness

While rebounding can't be considered as rigorous an aerobic activity as running or dance exercise, rope skipping can. For an activity that doesn't take you anywhere, skipping rope covers a lot of bases. (Skipping rope puts one foot on the ground at a time, alternately; jumping rope puts both feet on the ground simultaneously and is a bit more strenuous.)

When you skip or jump rope, you use muscles not only in your legs but also in your arms, back and shoulders. And the more muscles any given exercise incorporates, the more blood your heart has to pump— and the more oxygen your lungs must breathe to keep these muscles moving. It's for this reason that rope skipping compares so favorably with all other aerobic activities. When rope skipping was analyzed in laboratory experiments by Kenneth H. Cooper, M.D., 10 minutes' worth proved to be the fitness equivalent of jogging 1 mile in 10 to 12 minutes; cycling 3 miles in 9 to 12 minutes; swimming 350 yards in 6 to 8½ minutes; or playing 20 minutes of continuous handball, basketball or squash.

Jump with Joy—Not Pain

When skipping rope, wear sneakers or shoes with cushioned soles to protect your feet and absorb the shock, and don't jump on surfaces like concrete or asphalt. You can reduce the impact of a jump by jumping only high enough to clear the rope.

This exercise puts a lot of stress on your leg muscles and feet, so approach it as cautiously as if you were out for a long jog.

The experts say that a good way to get started on a rope-skipping program, in fact, is to alternate short bouts of jumping (anywhere from 30 seconds to a minute) with equal periods of rest until you become proficient (and conditioned) enough to jump for 20 minutes continuously.

That's a lot of exercise. And if you want to know more precisely the benefits that skipping rope can bestow, a study done with ten-year-old boys produced the following results: "Greater leg and knee strength, increased calf size, better jumping ability, faster running speed, greater agility and flexibility, broader shoulders and deeper chests and improved heart response." Not bad for an activity that need take you no further than your living room.

But how good is rope skipping at burning calories? Very good. Not quite as good as running, but still right up there with most other aerobic activities. For example, ten minutes of skipping rope (for someone weighing 150 pounds) burns approximately 100 calories. That's the equivalent of an equal amount of time spent jogging (at about a ten-minute-per-mile pace) or cycling (at about 13 miles an hour). Put another way, skipping rope burns about 10 calories a minute, for most people.

If you're the type who gets bored easily by exercise, at least while skipping rope you can watch TV or listen to music. You can even keep an eye on the kids, if need be.

Perhaps the most convenient aspect of all with skipping rope, though, is its portability. If you have to do a lot of traveling, it's certainly easier to pack a jump rope than a set of barbells or a stationary bicycle. It beats running because you needn't risk getting lost (or mugged) in a strange city. Just carry your trusty little jump rope with you and you can run your own minimarathon without ever leaving your hotel room.

There are ropes and there are ropes. You can spend as much as $12 for a super-duper leather job with wooden handles containing ball-bearings for easy turning—or you can cut yourself a length of clothesline and knot and tape the ends. Although what you decide to "swing" is up to you, each type of rope has certain features that you should be aware of.

Plastic "bead" ropes.   These are good for durability, if you opt for a relatively expensive rope; they're also good for control and jumping in the wind because of their greater weight.

Leather ropes.   This type is good for durability but difficult to control under windy conditions and not heavy enough for very fast or "trick" jumping.

"Rope" ropes.   These tend to wear out quickly (depending on the surface on which they're being used) and can be difficult to control if they're lightweight. They can also can burn your hands if not taped or equipped with wooden handles.

Heavyrope: Handle with Care

Kareem Abdul-Jabbar uses the Heavyrope for his workouts; should you?

Heavyrope is a weighted jump rope that its distributors say will condition both your muscles and your cardiovascular system.

"It almost ripped my arms out of the sockets," said one tester, a runner who also works out with weights. "I got shinsplints almost instantly after using it," said another tester who runs and does aerobic dance and circuit weight training. A third user, who is an aerobic-dance instructor and a runner, also felt the effects of Heavyrope on her shins.

So what gives? Is this a product to avoid? Not necessarily, says Budd Coates, a corporate fitness director and world-class marathoner.

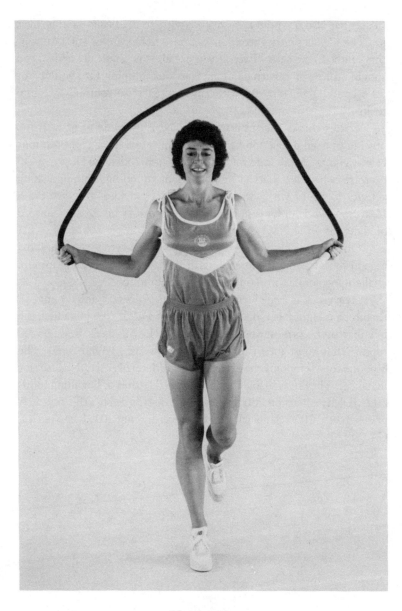

Heavyrope

Coates has also used the Heavyrope—with no ill effects—and he likes it. "The idea is pretty good; you just have to be careful and take your time with it," he says. "Even if you are already physically active, you should still go at it with caution. Start out jumping for about 15 or 20 seconds, then rest. As with any new exercise routine, ease into it slowly."

Coates thinks the testers quoted above probably went at it too quickly or used a rope too heavy for them (Heavyrope comes in four basic weights). More important, they may have added the Heavyrope to exercise schedules that had enough foot-pounding, shin-punishing activity to begin with. So it might be a good idea to *substitute* a Heavyrope workout for your usual run or aerobic-dance session, instead of adding it on.

On the plus side, all those who tried the Heavyrope thought it did a good job of strengthening the arm muscles and providing a more challenging aerobic workout than a plain jump rope.

Heavyrope is available in four weights (2, 3½, 5 and 6 pounds), each rope is eight feet long, and the cost is $34.95. As a guideline, the manufacturer says most women are comfortable with the 2- or 3½-pound ropes, while most men can handle the 3½- or 5-pound ropes. The 6-pound rope is for only the extremely fit athlete (like Abdul-Jabbar, for instance). They're available in sporting goods stores or by calling (800) ALL-JUMP, extension 260. Heavyrope is distributed by All-Pro Enterprises, Inc., 11050 Santa Monica Boulevard, Suite 201, Los Angeles, CA 90025.

Closet Stuffers You Can Use

Much of today's exercise equipment is handy and compact enough to fit neatly into a cubbyhole in the broom closet, on a small shelf in the garage, or even in a corner of your suitcase if you're a frequent traveler. Some items, as you'll learn in chapter 12, aren't worth a hoot when it comes to fitness, but some are well designed and easy to use and can help to enhance your total exercise program.

None of these really provides a complete enough workout to serve as the center of your fitness program. But they will assist you in zeroing in on a particular body part or fitness goal. Following are a few closet stuffers that we found interesting. (Check out your local sporting goods store for these exercise aids or others like them.)

Travel Exercisers

You're traveling on business and staying at a hotel that doesn't have a weight-training room. The only exercise you've had all day is shaking hands with clients, and you're dying to give your muscles a good workout. What can you do?

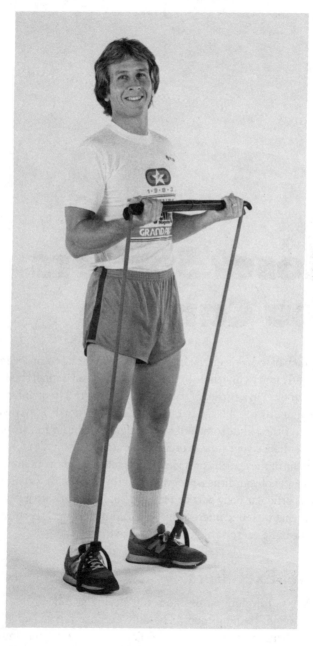

Lifeline Gym

Enter the travel exerciser. These portable muscle-resistance contraptions are lightweight and pack easily. But are these closet stuffers worth the money and trouble? Here's what we found out about two popular models.

The Lifeline Gym.   The Lifeline Gym provides resistance with a pliable cable that acts like a superstrong rubber band when you pull against it. When the cable is secured to something (like a door or your feet), you can use it to perform a variety of typical weight-training exercises. Lifeline also includes a bar with a groove into which the cable fits, so you can do arm exercises like presses and curls. For leg exercises and treadmill running, the gym features a belt that wraps around your foot or waist and is attached to the cable, which is then attached to a door.

Our testers generally liked the workout they got doing arm exercises with the cable and bar, although a few found it difficult to adjust the tension to their liking. Said one tester, "The tension tended to go from too little to too much." Another tester found the minimum tension adequate for some exercises but the maximum tension not tough enough for other exercises. (Since the cables come in different strengths, some of this problem could be resolved by exchanging the cable. However, our testers were using the proper cable strength for their weight and fitness levels.)

The testers found the leg exercises difficult and awkward to do because they couldn't get the strap to attach properly to the foot. Also, one tester said that because of the small size of many hotel rooms, she'd find it difficult to stretch Lifeline far enough to get the right tension for certain leg exercises.

Another tester, who travels frequently, pointed out that many hotel room doors lead into narrow passageways just inside the room. Because of this, he thought it might be difficult to perform some of the exercises near the door.

All of our testers found $40 a bit too pricey for this equipment. One tester said he'd once rigged a similar gym using inexpensive surgical tubing he'd purchased at a medical supply store or pharmacy. While it might not be as sophisticated or versatile as the Lifeline Gym, it would be less expensive.

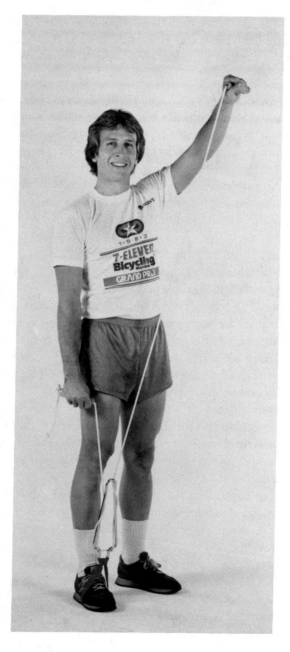

Gym In A Bag

The Gym In A Bag.   This is essentially a jump rope that is easily attached to a door through the use of a specially designed steel frame and strap. You can increase the resistance by looping the rope again and again through the steel frame. Your hand also acts as a resisting force: As you work out an arm or leg at one end of the rope, your control arm at the other end resists your exercising limb.

All of our testers found the Gym In A Bag more awkward to use than the Lifeline Gym. The rope tended to get tangled around its steel frame. Adjustments in tension were difficult to make and time-consuming. The rope was wobbly and difficult to control during an exercise.

Several of our exercisers said they had a hard time getting enough resistance to make the Gym In A Bag worth the trouble—they thought you could get nearly as good a workout doing your own calisthenics without the equipment. The Gym In A Bag retails for $19.95.

Medicine Balls: Making a Comeback

If you've ever seen a medicine ball, chances are it was being slammed into the abdomen of a grunting, hulking boxer, who was using it to develop superhuman stomach muscles. But you don't have to be the Incredible Hulk to benefit from the medicine ball—it's a great training tool for recreational athletes, too.

These large, weighted leather balls have been used by exercisers since the days of ancient Egypt and Greece. Medicine balls were a popular training device in the United States until World War II, when they were slowly displaced by calisthenics and heavy steel weight-training equipment. Now they're making a small but growing comeback among experts in the weight-training field as a complementary part of a strength-training regimen.

"The soft leather balls make a nice change from the hard steel of a weight room," says Jeff Miller, a strength and conditioning coach at United States International University, San Diego, California. Miller uses medicine balls as a regular part of athletes' training.

"Medicine balls train you to coordinate your body parts," says Charles C. Norelli, M.D., a specialist in physical medicine and rehabilitation. Dr. Norelli has used a medicine ball for years in his own fitness program. "For example, if you're throwing it, you can't just use your arm muscles; you're forced to use your entire body. That's good training for someone who's got to use his or her arm in sports—like a pitcher or a tennis player. Learning how to use your whole body instead of just your arm will help prevent strains in the arm muscles."

Dr. Norelli says that working out with a medicine ball teaches you to use your body correctly. "When you have to catch a heavy, weighted ball, you quickly learn how to do it without hurting your back or legs. You find out that you have to catch it close to your body's center of gravity. You have to bring your body to the ball—not lunge out beyond your reach to catch it."

Medicine ball exercises can be as varied as you want to make them. You can use the ball during your regular aerobics or calisthenics program. It makes a kind of resistive exercise without using weight machines.

Medicine balls can be difficult to locate. Since they went out of favor after World War II, they became scarce commodities. A sporting goods dealer could probably order one, however. For a moderately priced ball, Miller recommends the line made by Champion. They come in weights from 4 to 15 pounds and run from $10.50 to $26.00. A beginner would feel most comfortable with a 4- to 6-pound ball, says Miller. Later, you may want to purchase a heavier ball and keep the lighter one for warm-ups. Champion Medicine Balls are made by BSN/Champion Corporation, P.O. Box 7726, Dallas, TX 75209 (800-527-7510; in Texas, 800-442-3451).

A more expensive but extremely well made medicine ball recommended by Miller is the Lineaus Medicine Ball. Made by a group of medicine ball aficionados, these balls come in weights of 6 to 16 pounds and cost about $125. (So-called heavy balls, which are smaller in diameter, cost $75 and range in weight from 3½ to 7½ pounds.) The makers of the Lineaus Medicine Balls have also produced a book of medicine ball conditioning routines. For more information on both items, contact Lineaus Medicine Balls, Route 1, Box 159, Kyle, TX 78640 (512-398-7513).

The Kyga Stick: Compact and Versatile

The Kyga Stick is a pretty amazing feat of design. Contained in one extremely small tote bag (6 by 6 by 12 inches) are 20 pounds of free weights, a variable-resistance rope that enables you to perform traditional weight-lifting exercises and straps that allow you to do leg exercises with the weights, plus a connector and an extender that further increase the system's versatility. The free weights are designed as cylinders that fit inside each other. There are ten, in varying weights that can be used in different combinations.

Two testers that we recruited said that the rope gave enough resistance to simulate a workout you'd perform on weight machines. Neither felt, however, that someone who already worked out in a gym would give it up for the Kyga Stick. If you didn't have access to weight-lifting equipment, though, it would be a compact system that would not take up a lot of space in your home.

The Kyga Stick may be compact, but it certainly isn't portable. That was the assessment of our third tester, who works out in aerobics classes. Our other two testers agreed with her. The bag in which the Kyga system is contained looks small, but it is far too heavy to carry any distance. It would be impractical to take on a business trip, they felt.

So, all in all, the testers gave the Kyga Stick a mixed review. Admiration for its design and general comfort was offset by complaints about its other features. If you like gadgetry and don't mind some assembly and disassembly time, the Kyga Stick may be for you. If you have easy access to a gym and like to get your workout over with a minimum of fuss, you may not like this device.

The Kyga Stick is available for $89.95 from Kyga, Inc., P.O. Box 24325, Denver, CO 80224.

Other Worthwhile Items

Here are a few more closet stuffers that can help to round out your workout.

Handgrips.   People who work out sometimes concentrate on a few muscle areas and ignore many others. Often, they end up looking trim and toned in places like the stomach and out of kilter somewhere else. The purpose of Handgrips is to develop the forearm and strengthen the wrist and finger grip. Making such muscles stronger can probably help your racquetball or tennis game, since strong muscles translate into more endurance. Even hauling luggage or getting grocery bags out of the trunk may not seem like such an overwhelming task.

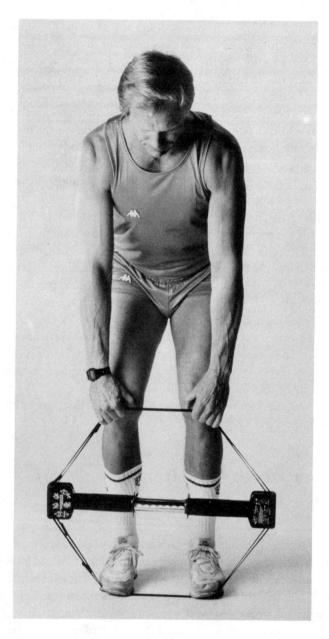

Bullworker

Bullworkers.   The Bullworker X5, made by the Margrace Corporation, can be used to build strength and muscular endurance. This versatile piece of equipment, the latest in a long line of Bullworker products, will perform 42 different exercises that strengthen the upper and lower body. It's lightweight and completely portable— ideal for traveling.

Exercise mats.   They sure beat the living room rug. One particular mat, the six-foot Aerobics Mat by Sentinel Fitness Products, absorbs body shock well, is impervious to perspiration and folds in half for easy toting to those exercise classes away from home. This mat is available at most good sporting goods stores for about $48.

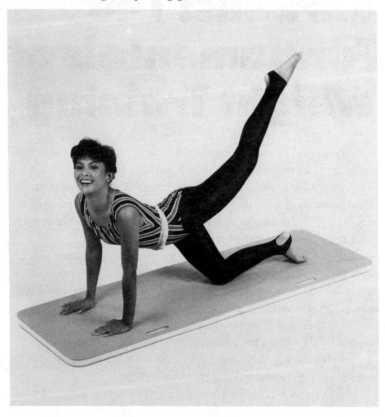

Aerobics Mat

Dumbbells and Barbells: The Fundamentals of Weight Training

Many people picture weight lifters as huge hulks in love with their bodies or as Olympic titans who heft barbells that would give King Kong a hard time. Well, if that's your image of weight training, you might want to change it. Lifting weights isn't just for weirdos and supermen—it's for *anyone.* That is, anyone who wants either to get in shape or to improve on the fitness he's already achieved.

To start a weight-training program, the first equipment you are going to need is a set of weights—obviously. According to experienced weight lifters, both pro and amateur, a set of barbells and dumbbells gives the best results.

A barbell is the big weight bar, the kind that you lift with two hands. Dumbbells are the small weights, the ones you can lift single-handed. By having both dumbbells and barbells, you'll be able to develop more muscles by doing more movements.

All Olympic standard barbells are seven feet long. The kind you'll probably buy will be five to six feet long. The central bar that holds the weights should have a loose-fitting sleeve that sits around the middle of the bar. Collars on each side of the bar secure the weights to the bar.

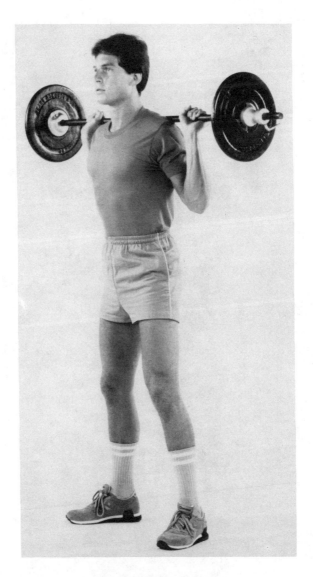

Metal Barbell

For the exercises, you'll need two dumbbells. These are usually about 18 inches long. Their construction is similar to that of the larger barbell.

Steve Jarrell, an experienced weight lifter, recommends having at least 90 pounds of plates. (Plates are the circular, weighted slabs that

(continued on page 48)

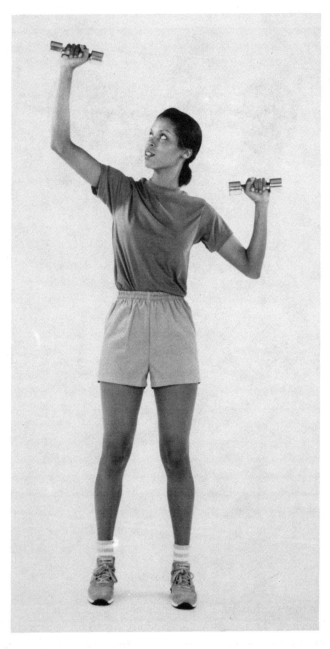

Chrome Dumbbells

A Sample Weight-Training Program

Week	Session 1: Heavy Weight Day	Session 2: Light Weight Day	Session 3: Medium Weight Day
1	10 repetitions of each exercise, at the maximum weight load you can lift 10 times	10 repetitions of each exercise at a much lighter weight than your maximum 10-repetition load (about 70–80% of maximum)	10 repetitions of each exercise at a somewhat lighter weight than your maximum 10-repetition load (about 80–90% of maximum)
2 & 3	repeat week 1, session 1	repeat week 1, session 2	repeat week 1, session 3
4	5 repetitions of each exercise at the maximum weight load you can lift 5 times	5 repetitions of each exercise at a much lighter weight than your maximum 5-repetition load (about 70–80% of maximum)	5 repetitions of each exercise at a somewhat lighter weight than your maximum 5-repetition load (about 80–90% of maximum)
5 & 6	repeat week 4, session 1	repeat week 4, session 2	repeat week 4, session 3
7	3 repetitions of each exercise at the maximum weight load you can lift 3 times	3 repetitions of each exercise at a much lighter weight than your maximum 3-repetition load (about 70–80% of maximum)	3 repetitions of each exercise at a somewhat lighter weight than your maximum 3-repetition load (about 80–90% of maximum)
8 & 9	repeat week 7, session 1	repeat week 7, session 2	repeat week 7, session 3

SOURCE: John J. Garhammer, Ph.D., International Maxachievement Institutes, Long Beach, California.
NOTE: This program can be integrated into a circuit-weight or any other series of strength-training exercises. Once you complete it, begin again, but incorporate some different exercises into your routine. If you can, use a variety of free weights and weight machines. All of these factors vary your strength-training diet and keep your body guessing, which is what keeps it working.

A Barbell Safety Tip

For safety's sake, before you pick up a barbell with weights on it, make sure that the weights are securely attached. The collars that hold on the weighted plates should be screwed on as tight as possible. Otherwise, you run the risk of having them slide off the bar and land on you, your floor, your furniture or whatever else is nearby—with unpleasant results.

attach to the bars.) Most sets available in stores are the 110-pound "basic sets" that include 90 pounds of plates. The most common plate sizes are 2½, 5, 10 and 25 pounds.

When you go to buy weights, you'll probably have a choice between metal plates and plastic plates filled with sand. The metal plates are more expensive and noisier when you lift them up and clang them down. Their advantage over the cheaper plastic weights is that they will last much longer. The plastic weights will eventually wear out.

The plastic weights usually cost about $35 to $40; the metal weights retail for about $70. When you think about it, much of this equipment is less expensive than many running shoes! And the weights, even if you use them every day, will outlast the shoes by a decade.

Weight Training for Travelers

If you hate missing workouts but don't feel like lugging 5-pound dumbbells around in your suitcase, you might try Travel Weights. They're collapsible and weigh only 2.2 pounds— fill them with water or sand to make them accommodate your personal exercise preferences. Travel weights are available in several colors, come with a separate carrying case, and retail for around $37. Look for them at sporting goods stores.

Nautilus and Universal Machines: Easy-Does-It Weight Training

Ten years ago, the average weight-training club had all the charm of a steel mill. The floor was littered with barbells, many of them so loaded with weight that just removing enough pounds to make them liftable for the new user was a workout in itself. There was also a din of clanking as exercisers banged dumbbells together over their heads or chests, and reverberating *Booms!* as power lifters dropped hundreds of pounds of metal on ancient wooden platforms.

But such scenes are rapidly disappearing, as many gyms convert to either the Universal or Nautilus system of resistance training.

One Machine, Many Uses

The Universal Gym is by far the simpler of the two. When you work out with the Universal, you push or pull against bars connected to levers or pulleys, which in turn are attached to stacked weights. To change the resistance, all you need to do is remove a steel pin from one hole and insert it in another. And there is no chance at all of dropping 90 pounds on your kneecap, because the weights are confined in the "body" of the mechanism.

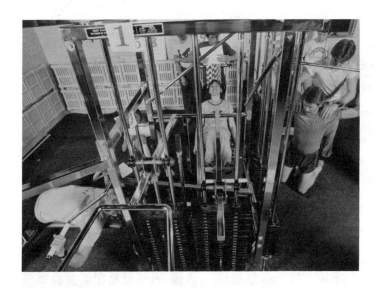

Universal Gym

The Nautilus Way

The Nautilus approach is radically different—and looks it. A Nautilus gym may have from 6 to 8 to as many as 20 specialized machines, each designed to work out specific sets of muscles. Looking like a cross between ultramodern furniture and medical devices, a roomful of Nautilus-type equipment can easily cost as much as two or three Cadillacs. But its advocates say it's worth it.

The biomechanical philosophy of Nautilus equipment is that while barbells and the like are simply heavy, clumsy weights, Nautilus equipment is specifically designed to accommodate human musculature through a wide range of motion.

Let's say that you want to give the pectoral muscles of your upper chest a good workout using dumbbells. A popular exercise for doing this consists of lying flat on a padded bench, with a dumbbell in each

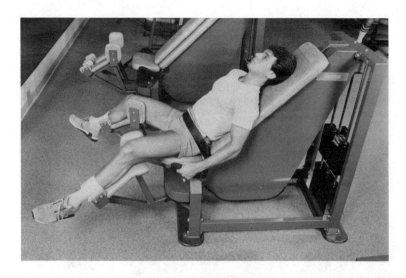

Nautilus Abductor/Adductor Machine

hand. Just getting yourself into this position can be awkward and
stressful. Then, with your arms slightly bent, the weights are lowered
to the sides until they are just a few inches below the level of the bench.
At that point, the stress on your muscles (and joints) is relatively great,
and the effort of moving them up again is very great. But once your
arms have reached about a 45-degree angle, the effort diminishes
rapidly, reaching the null point as the two weights meet over your chest.
The resistance diminishes so rapidly, in fact, that the dumbbells often
smash together. The result is an unbalanced exercise.

To perform essentially the same exercise with Nautilus equipment, you don't have to load any dumbbells or get them in position for
lying down on a bench. All you do is stand with your back against a
machine, press the inner side of your forearms against two large pads
on opposite sides of your chest, and then move your arms inward until
the two pads touch each other. That sounds very undramatic (and
quiet, too!). But what's happening behind you is pretty exciting. There,
a system of cams and chains is performing automatic adjustments to
provide a constant level of resistance to your chest muscles throughout
the entire range of the exercise, from beginning to end. The result is
more balanced development of strength and muscle mass. And, as with
the Universal Gym, resistance levels can be changed in seconds.

In many ways then—including muscle development, safety and convenience—Nautilus seems to be a superior method of resistance training. However, unless you have a very large spare room and a very

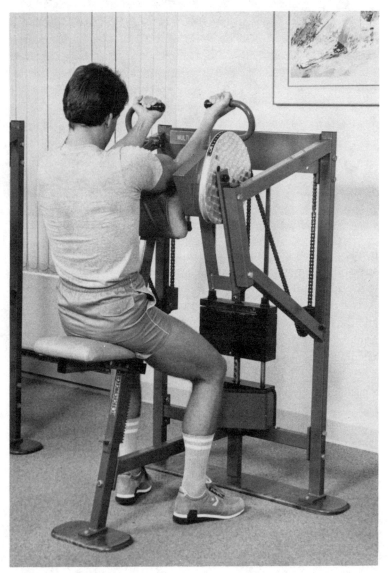

Nautilus Double-Arm Machine

large bank account, you will have to go to a club to use Nautilus equipment. Barbells and dumbbells (or free weights, as they're called) can be purchased for home use for a fraction of the price of Nautilus equipment and stashed in a closet when they're not being used. So in some ways, they are actually *more* convenient.

Home Nautilus Machines

The Nautilus Low-Back and Abdominal machines are not new; you may have seen or used them at your health club. But now Nautilus has begun selling these machines in scaled-down versions for use in the home.

We consulted a doctor who specializes in back problems, an exercise physiologist, a physical therapist and a doctor who specializes in rehabilitative medicine. One of the four had actually used the machines. The other three were familiar with the products through advertising claims made by Nautilus. Here's what they thought.

The Low-Back Machine. Nautilus claims that this machine will stretch and strengthen what they call "your back's critical muscles—the erector spinae," which are the muscles in your lower back. You sit at almost a right angle and push the pad behind your upper back until your body is straight. Our experts had three primary reservations about the machine.

First, the erector spinae muscles are the least important of the four major muscle groups that are crucial to back health. Much more important to exercise are the abdominals, the hip muscles and the side muscles. Although some of our experts thought the Low-Back Machine might also work the abdominals somewhat, others thought it wouldn't be enough to really strengthen them.

Second, the lower back muscles are probably the most vulnerable and least understood of all the muscles that support the spine. None of our experts would recommend this machine to people with back problems.

And finally, even if you were in great shape and had no back problems, our experts wondered why you would want a machine in your home that exercises such a limited area of the body. If you're trying to prevent back problems later on, you need to exercise all four of the muscle groups mentioned above, not just one.

The Abdominal Machine.   This machine operates in just the opposite way from the Low-Back Machine. The pads are flush against your chest, and to operate the machine, you push downward toward your feet and contract your abdominals.

Our experts felt that there is no question that this machine does what it says it will do, which is strengthen the abdominals. However, most of them also felt that a good Sit-Up, if done properly without anchoring your feet, would give you the same benefits as this machine.

All of them questioned whether this machine is a good buy for the home—not only because you can do Sit-Ups for free but also because the machine once again works on only one set of muscles. If it's available at your health club, however, go ahead and use it. But be sure to exercise your other back-support muscles within your regular exercise regimen.

The Low-Back Machine retails for $435, and the Abdominal Machine retails for $485. For more information about them, contact Nautilus, P.O. Box 1119, Lake Helen, FL 32744 (800-874-8941).

A Step-by-Step Guide to Wrist and Ankle Weights

Wrist and ankle weights have been around in gyms and training programs for ages, but light weights—not more than a couple of pounds each—are a relatively new concept in aerobic workouts. They're being touted as the safest, most effective way to supplement aerobic exercise. Trainers and coaches are incorporating them into running and walking programs. Books and videos are already appearing. Classes especially designed around the use of light weights are cropping up all over the country.

So light weights are catching on. But are they effective workout enhancers? And, more important, will they increase the benefit of your workout without increasing your risk of injury? Here's what we found out.

Hand Weights: Are They Safe? Do They Work?

It was a marriage made in heaven, some said. Take a simple set of light weights, teach people how to use them in pumping motions that exercise the upper body, and then combine them with a running or walking program for a total body workout.

That's exactly what Leonard Schwartz, M.D., a Pittsburgh psychiatrist and fitness specialist, did in his first book, *Heavyhands: The Ultimate Exercise System.* People took to it in droves and soon it was common to see exercisers out on the road clutching weights and pumping as they sped along.

Have hand weights caused any major problems or injuries to users in their first few years of big popularity? We called a number of exercise and human performance labs around the country, as well as the American College of Sports Medicine and the National Strength and Conditioning Association. Their answers: no major problems reported yet. Because the weights are so light, they shouldn't pose a threat to joints or muscles.

As a way to improve and enhance aerobic capacity (and burn more calories in the process), hand weights get high marks. "The extra work that the muscles have to perform, even with very light weights, fatigues them more quickly, which increases the workload on the cardiovascular system," says Linda Shelton, an exercise physiologist from Thousand Oaks, California, and the national training coordinator for the Aerobics and Fitness Association of America (AFAA). A weighted workout, she adds, is often just what is needed to kick a person over the aerobic "plateau" to a higher level of fitness.

Light weights are also good news for anyone wishing to burn a few extra calories and reduce body fat. For instance, explains Thomas Pipes, an exercise physiologist and director of the National Institute of Human Fitness in Diamond Springs, California, "If you normally burn 200 calories in a regular aerobic workout, you will burn 230 calories with the addition of half-pound weights on each wrist."

Increased muscle strength is another benefit of light-weight workouts. In a six-week study of college-age women, those who used half-pound weights in their aerobic workouts three times a week gained 50 percent more upper-body strength than those who worked without weights. These figures may seem impressive, but, as Pipes points out, "most regular aerobic workouts do not result in a significant increase in upper-body strength."

The added resistance of a weighted workout can also lead to marked muscle definition that is not usually possible to achieve in a

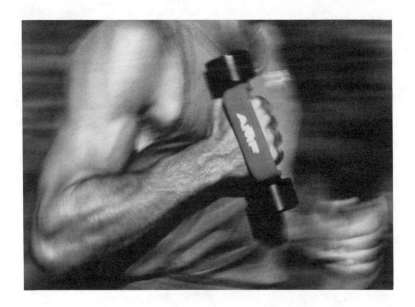

Heavyhands

regular aerobics program. Leora Myers, a competitive body builder and exercise consultant who teaches a light-weight program called Super Shaping in San Francisco, finds that women nowadays want the extra definition that the weights can provide. "When I first started my program, the women in my classes weren't sure they wanted that extra muscle," she says. "But it's catching on now—my classes are packed!"

They're also a good idea for people with orthopedic problems, says Bryant Stamford, Ph.D., of the Exercise Physiology Laboratory at the University of Louisville, Kentucky. "If you're walking four miles in an hour and you want to increase your workload—but jogging is not an alternative—then you could add hand weights instead."

There is a myriad of different styles of light weights to choose from. Handheld weights, such as the popular Heavyhands and GraFar's Space Weights, are fine as long as you don't grip them too tightly; this creates undue muscle tension and restricts blood flow, according to one expert. The strap-on variety for wrists and ankles should fasten securely so they don't slip; loose weights can result in a lack of control, warns Shelton.

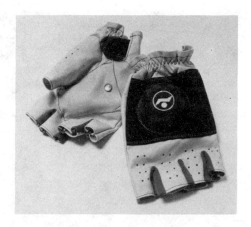

Weighted Gloves

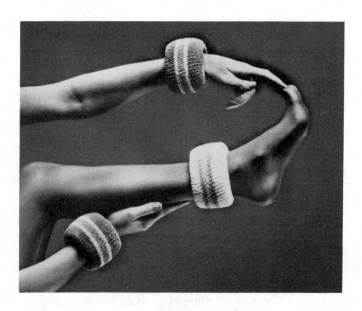

Wrist and Ankle Weights

Weighted, stretchy bands help to eliminate the slipping problem. Weighted gloves have also become popular alternatives to handheld and wrist weights.

Ankle Weights: Handle with Care

There's some good news and some bad news for those of you who strap on ankle weights. If you're using them while running, you could be asking for injuries. But if you're using them in a strengthening regimen, they're a fine way to add a little more resistance to your own body's.

That's the assessment of John Pagliano, D.P.M., a Long Beach, California, sports podiatrist who specializes in running injuries, and Ronald Fell, Ph.D., an exercise physiologist from the Exercise Physiology Laboratory at the University of Louisville.

What's wrong with using weights for running? "The weights put stress on your joints—a stress they're not used to," Dr. Pagliano says. "When you run, you're stressing joints anyway. The added weight simply compresses your knee, hip, lower back and foot joints even more."

For the short term, adding extra weight to your legs may cause you only minor problems, like tendon and ligament strains or muscle pulls. But later on in life, that added stress on your joints could give you arthritic problems, says Dr. Pagliano.

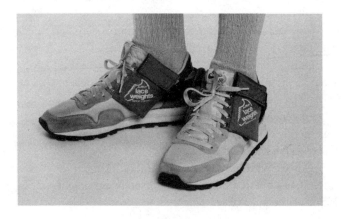

Lace Weights

"The problem with joggers using ankle weights is that they try to go out and run their usual mileage," says Dr. Fell. "That can be dangerous for the heart as well as cause orthopedic problems. Rather than using ankle weights, they would do better to increase their mileage to improve fitness."

Dr. Fell says lightweight (they start at one pound per foot), lace-on ankle weights would probably be okay if you cut back your running mileage. Anything over one pound, however, should be avoided.

So give your legs a break when you run. Save heavy ankle weights for your leg lifts and abdominal strengthening exercises.

Yet, because ankle weights can increase your heart's workout, Dr. Fell thinks they're probably a good option for people who *walk* for exercise. "If you can't run because of some orthopedic or other problem, the weights could enhance your caloric expenditure and increase your aerobic fitness." To see if weights really would make a difference

When Not to Use Weights

Generally, light weights should not be used during the warm-up or cool-down segment of a workout.

Ankle weights should *never* be used during high-impact workouts—while running or jumping in an aerobics class, for example.

Very fast movements that rely on momentum, like rapid arm circles, should not be done with weights.

Don't use weights on a limb that has been injured, except in a rehabilitation program supervised by a physician or therapist.

Anyone with known cardiovascular disease, a history of high blood pressure, or increased risk of heart attack or hypertension should not use weights.

Anyone with muscle strains, joint or ligament injuries, tendinitis or bursitis should refrain from using weights until a doctor or therapist okays their use.

when you walk, Dr. Fell suggests that you compare your pulse while walking without weights to your pulse when you are using them.

Dr. Fell would not recommend using ankle weights during the bouncing and jumping segments of aerobics classes. "With all that jumping and twisting, the extra weight could cause your foot to hit the ground harder. You'd have a lot of the same problems joggers do," he says.

Still, both Dr. Fell and Dr. Pagliano feel that ankle weights could complement calisthenics or other strengthening programs. "You'll work the muscles really well, and that's fine," says Dr. Pagliano. Ankle weights come in almost as many varieties as wrist and hand weights; your job is to make sure the pair you wear fits snugly.

Computer Fitness

Want to be more scientific in your approach to fitness? Then you might want to try using a monitor that displays your heart rate as you exercise. These monitors use sensors to find the pulse in your fingertip, earlobe or chest. And many experts claim they're far more accurate than trying to use your hand to take the pulse at your neck. In contrast, these monitors leave you free to concentrate on your exercise form. Moreover, they keep you honest. You can't kid yourself about working hard when the pulse monitor says otherwise.

Which One Do I Buy?

There are two types of units: the heart rate monitor, which picks up the heart's electrical impulses with electrodes, and the pulse monitor, which detects and records with infrared light the pulsation of blood coursing through the blood vessels. In terms of accuracy, neither type has an advantage: both receive signals from the heart at approximately the same time. Individual units, however, are another story, since their computer circuitry and design all contribute to overall efficiency. In other words, what makes one unit superior to another is the nature of the components, rather than where the monitor picks up your pulse. In our tests, most of the pulse monitors compared quite favorably to an electrocardiograph (ECG) unit, which hospitals use for heart measurements.

Our advice is to shop carefully. Since exercises like cycling are unpredictable, you'll need a monitor that can withstand anything from a downpour to a pothole. You'll also want to consider the unit's price and weight, and whether it's easy to use and understand. The prices are dropping drastically. If you've shopped for pulse monitors in the past with little success, don't give up yet.

Finger-Sensor Units

We found the finger-sensor units we tested to be lightweight, durable and easy to use—just attach the sensor clamp to your finger. But there are a few precautions: don't press your finger too hard against the clamp's sensor crystal, or the unit will break. Also, make sure you're reading your pulse properly. Should the manufacturer require you to attach the sensor to the left hand, keep in mind that the pulse there is stronger than in the right hand.

The Pulse-Tach CPS4. This was the smallest unit we tested. Two inches long, the monitor has a single integrated circuit chip that calibrates pulse, time of day and exercise time. To use it, slip the tip of your left index finger along the groove in the back of the unit.

As the small blood vessels in your finger expand with each heartbeat, the light is reflected back to the sensor, where your pulse is recorded and flashed in digital numbers on a small screen in front. Push the "pulse" button and your pulse will appear every ten seconds. Tap the "pulse" button again and the computer will average your heartbeat every four seconds. The latter is particularly useful when you don't want to wait every ten seconds for your pulse. You can also use the built-in timer to determine your recovery rate. Exercisers will find the Pulse-Tach's greatest asset is its size.

You probably won't be able to keep the Pulse-Tach attached to your finger the entire time you exercise, but it can be useful for intermittent checks on your heart. Be sure to steady your hand before taking your

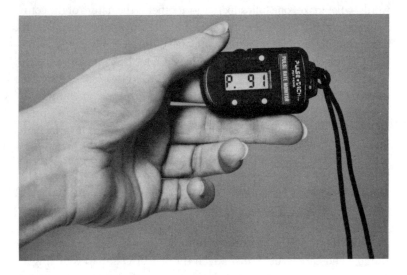

Pulse-Tach CPS4

pulse: movement gives an erratic reading. One advantage of the Pulse-Tach is that your heartbeats are displayed in black digital numbers that you can read in any type of weather.

The Pulse-Tach monitor comes in either the finger-clamp model or as a Pulse-Tach wristwatch. Both units have the same type of circuitry, but you need two hands to operate the wristwatch.

One drawback: don't count on using the Pulse-Tach in cold weather. As your finger becomes cold, it becomes more difficult for the unit to detect a pulse. Above 32°F, however, it seems to function just fine.

The Pulse-Tach CPS4 weighs 0.75 ounce, including its power source of two 1.5-volt watch batteries, and has a 90-day warranty. It is distributed by DNA Medical, Inc., 391 Chipeta Way, Suite B, Salt Lake City, UT 84108; the price is $69.95. The Pulse-Tach Watch, distributed by The Sharper Image, 300 Broadway, Suite 28, San Francisco, CA 94133, costs $99.00 plus $3.50 for delivery.

The Genesis Exercise Computer.   This monitor has a number of functions. Worn like a wristwatch, it has a time-of-day display; a pulse monitor; a calculator that programs your preexercise pulse plus upper and lower heart rate; an audio alert that sounds when you're working too hard or not hard enough; an exercise timer that logs how long you've exercised in your target zone; and a variable speed metronome that helps you set your cadence.

Just strap the computer around your wrist, fasten the band and attach the sensor and cord to your left index finger. If you're cycling, you'll still be able to brake, but don't squeeze the finger clamp too hard, or you'll break the crystal inside. Unlike the Pulse-Tach, the Genesis sensor contains a microphonelike device that measures the blood circulation with sound waves.

The Genesis Exercise Computer is available from Biometric Systems, Inc., 4040 Del Ray Avenue, Marina Del Ray, CA 90291 and costs $159.95. It weighs 2.3 ounces, including its power source of two 1.5-volt batteries, and has a one-year warranty.

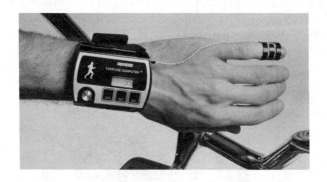

Genesis Exercise Computer

Earlobe Sensors

Earlobe sensors rated quite high in accuracy, and since you can keep your head steadier than your hand, there was less of a problem with movement and a fluctuating heart rate.

The Amerec PM-110 Pulse Meter. With its compact carrying case, long cord and earlobe sensor, this monitor looks a little like a transistor radio.

Cycling seems to be the sport best suited for the Amerec's design, since a helmet will keep the earlobe sensor firmly in place. It is a little harder to keep the clamp in place while jogging. The sensor light must face the back of the earlobe for accurate pulse readings: we found that, when used properly, the Amerec matched the hospital's ECG machine nearly beat for beat.

This unit can take a lot of work out of your training program—at least when it comes to calculating numbers. The Amerec has a time-of-day display and a timer; you can also see your pulse and time displayed at four-second intervals.

The Amerec was convenient and lightweight, and it withstood punishment. No amount of wiggling or frame-shaking could tumble the monitor bracket, once it was properly installed. Moreover, the ear sensor didn't slip once, even with some rigorous head shaking.

The Amerec PM-110 weighs 12.6 ounces (including batteries and bracket), operates on size AA batteries and has a one-year warranty. It comes with a bracket and screws and is easy to install. The unit, which sells for $129, is distributed by the Amerec Corporation, P.O. Box 3825, Bellevue, WA 98009.

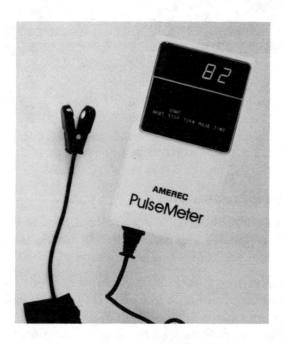

Amerec Pulse Meter

Chest Monitors

These heart monitors use electrodes that strap to your chest to detect your heart rate.

The PE 2000 Sport Tester.   This model uses advanced radio technology to beam your pulse onto a small wristwatch monitor. The monitor picks up the signal from a rubber chest strap that contains electrodes similar to those used with ECG machines. There are no wires, so you have complete freedom of movement.

The Sport Tester provides information on regular time, elapsed time and average pulse, as well as a moment-to-moment readout on where the heart is headed. "I was surprised to find out that my pulse wasn't as high as I thought it was when I did hill work," said one tester. "I also found out that I probably needed to give myself more time to cool down—I thought I was doing it long enough, but my pulse was still elevated."

The Sport Tester is made in Finland and is distributed by AMF American, Inc., 200 American Avenue, Jefferson, IA 50129 (800-247-3978). It costs $250.

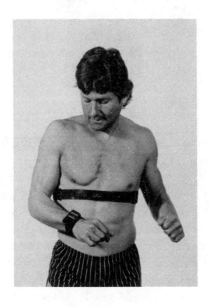

PE 2000 Sport Tester

The Coach.   A complete fitness computer as well as a heart rate monitor, The Coach works differently from the Sport Tester. It also uses a chest strap with electrodes, but there's a wire that runs from the strap to the minicomputer, which clips to your waistband (or to the front of your bike if you're a cyclist). The readout runs along the top of the monitor, so you look down at your belt to read it.

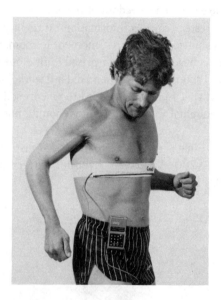

The Coach

"While the cloth chest strap made it more comfortable than the other pulse monitor, I found it unnatural to be looking at my waistband all the time," commented one tester. The wire wasn't an annoyance, however.

The Coach has all the same features as the Sport Tester—and these got the same high marks—but it also offers much more. It will tell you the number of calories you've burned; how fit you are; the number of miles you've covered; the speed at which you've traveled; and the number of steps you've taken. It is made by Biotechnology, Inc., 6924 Northwest 46th Street, Miami, FL 33166 (800-327-1033), and costs $199.95.

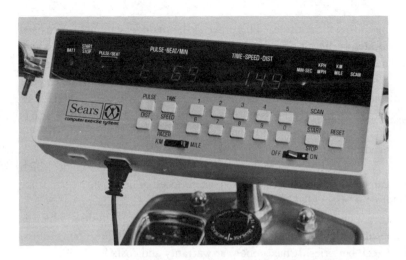

Sears Digital Electronic Exercise/Pulse Monitor

The Sears Monitor

The Sears Digital Electronic Exercise/Pulse Monitor is designed to be used on a regular bicycle or exercise bike, and it comes with more optional features than many of the other units we tested. The computer can record both upper and lower heart rate; target distance, time and mileage; actual mileage in kilometers or miles; the time; and your pulse. This can be an asset for those who take their training seriously. While doing intervals, for instance, you can preprogram your target time and distance. A beeper will sound when you reach your goal. You can also use the Sears monitor to train for endurance; just set the time and your target zone, and a buzzer will sound when you've exceeded your limits.

The other advantage to this pulse monitor is that it displays both your heart rate and the time at the same moment on two different screens. This saves you a lot of trouble, especially during interval training when you want to know both your pulse and time.

In fact, this unit has only one glaring flaw—the console is simply too big! It measures 12 inches long and weighs over two pounds. Its length makes it difficult to mount on a road bike, as the manufacturer points out in the directions: "This pulse monitor can be used on a standard outdoor bicycle, but some difficulty could be experienced in mounting the console." This proved to be an understatement. You need to attach the mounting brackets to *each side* of the monitor, which means you need a span of about 14 inches between your handlebars. As a result, you have to hammer and prod the brackets into the smaller space on your bike. You can't afford to be sloppy in installation, since the whole thing can fall off unless you're careful. But once the brackets are firmly in place, you'll find it's a sturdy companion, barely shaking even over some rough-and-tumble terrain.

The only other problem with the Sears model is its weight, which can be a burden when trying to pick up speed or negotiate a turn, since it does affect bike handling.

The Sears Digital Electronic Exercise/Pulse Monitor, which is available from Sears, weighs 2.2046 pounds, including four alkaline C-cell batteries. It has a one-year warranty and costs $199.99.

Monitoring Your Stride

Some gizmos are designed simply to keep track of how far you walk—or how hard you run.

Pedometer: A walker's companion.   Setting a mileage goal for walking and sticking to it—that's not always so easy. A pedometer helps you out. Just measure your stride toe to toe, then clip the pocket-size device onto your waist. A small pendulum inside clocks your miles as it ticks off each stride. Pedometers run about $15 and come with a digital or clock face. Just remember that a pedometer will be only as stable and accurate as your stride.

The RunAlert.   The RunAlert is a matchbox-size monitor that you clip to your running shorts. It contains a meter that measures how hard your foot strikes the ground. Since a heavy foot-strike is believed to be the source of many running injuries, the idea behind RunAlert is to make you aware of how hard you run and to remind you to run more efficiently. A range of settings allows you to preselect the impact with which you want to hit the ground. If you exceed that impact, a beeper sounds.

The concept is a good one, but the runners who tested this product for us had one complaint: It was very difficult to get the beeper to stop,

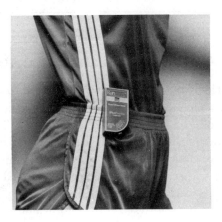

RunAlert

unless they were running on a completely flat, unchanging surface. Since most runners spend some time on hills and probably change surfaces a few times (from grass to a roadway, for example), the beeper can drive you nuts.

"I think there may be a place for it, but it hasn't come far enough along in technology," believes Budd Coates, a world-class marathoner who competed in the Olympic trials in 1984. Coates tried the RunAlert and found that it had limited use. "If you're running downhill, for example, you naturally hit the ground harder. If you start trying to run softer to get that beeper to stop, you might wind up doing more harm than good to your muscles when they're in that position."

Coates thinks that the RunAlert would be fine for interval training on a track. It would allow you to monitor the fatigue caused by speedwork and its effects on form and foot-strike.

Fitness instructor Eileen Portz also used the RunAlert on her runs and found that the beeper drove her crazy. "I think I run pretty efficiently—I've never suffered from a lot of injuries, yet it was very hard to get the beeper to stop, even on the heaviest setting," she observed. Portz could get it to stop on a flat surface, but as soon as she picked up speed, changed surface or encountered a hill, the beeper started.

We asked Mike Chan, president of RunTronics, the firm that produces the RunAlert, about some of the complaints we were hearing. He said he'd been hearing some of the same complaints himself. "I think the RunAlert is definitely more for people interested in avoiding

Computerized Workouts:
A Glimpse of the Future

After a hard day at the office, you head for your health club, where you insert your computer fitness disk into a small computer hooked up to special exercise equipment. The disk programs the computer to adapt the equipment to the best speed, range of motion and weight resistance for your needs (which can be either strength training or aerobic endurance work). It guides you through your planned exercise program while the computer screen shows you information on your progress, as measured against your past performance. The screen also indicates how many calories you're burning. While resting between sets, you can check stock market closing prices and catch the news.

Sound fantastic? This combination of computer technology and exercise science exists in the Ariel Computerized Exercise Machine, which is already being used by the U.S. Olympic Committee and exercise labs to train athletes. Its creator, Gideon Ariel, Ph.D., developed the system to be used by the Olympic athletes he trains at his own Coto Research Center in Coto de Caza, California.

But Dr. Ariel thinks that one day it will be used by insurance companies to certify fitness discounts for business executives or by large hotel chains that cater to executive clients. You'd simply bring your computer program from your home health club and plug into the hotel's equipment.

Dr. Ariel, whose background includes both biomechanics and computers, is a former Olympic discus thrower. His equipment has already been purchased by almost 200 schools and fitness centers, including Harvard University and the Massachusetts Institute of Technology. But we don't think it's something you'll want to consider yet for your home gym. The price tag for the setup is $16,500.

injuries than for those who simply want to run fast." Chan said that the beeper goes off when you're running on hills because that puts a lot of stress on the body. He advises runners to walk or run slowly at those times. He also said that changing from grass to concrete, for example, will definitely set it off for the same reason—the concrete creates greater stress.

Chan said that he tells experienced runners to set the device at a point where it beeps about once every 10 to 15 steps. "Then, as you get tired, it might start beeping more. That's an indication that your form is starting to break down and you're starting to hit the ground too hard. Maybe it's time to end your run if you want to avoid injuring yourself."

Beginning runners may find it more of a challenge to get the device to stop beeping, said Chan. But he feels it may help them develop better running habits right from the start.

A booklet comes with the RunAlert that teaches you how to use it and offers advice on how to soften your foot's impact on the ground by wearing good shoes or running on forgiving surfaces. The RunAlert is available for $29.95 from RunTronics, Inc., P.O. Box 391143, Mountain View, CA 94039.

Home Sweet Home Gym

The best thing about a home gym is that you are *home.* What could be more convenient? And if you've ever been tempted in the past to skip a workout, gone is the excuse that you don't feel like getting into your car and driving somewhere to exercise.

What's more, in the long run, a home gym will pay for itself in time and money saved. There's no more commuting to and from your health club in traffic. You don't spend time waiting in line to use a machine. You aren't dishing out hundreds of dollars a year to maintain your health club membership; instead, you have a "membership that never expires." And, if you've chosen your equipment wisely, you still get a complete workout.

If you've never looked into the possibility of a home gym, you might be surprised that you can get a health club workout with all the conveniences of home. To demonstrate, we assembled the three "mini-gyms" shown in the photos on the following pages. We selected equipment that is durable, convenient to set up and use, and safe to use alone or with others. Because budgets for fitness equipment vary, we selected three price ranges.

For as little as $70, you can get a 110-pound set of free weights. Add a padded bench with a rack and you increase the number of exercise options. With your own resistance weight machine, such as the Universal Power-Pak, you can lift heavier weights without the need for a spotter, as would be the case with heavier free weights.

In each grouping we've also included an option for indoor aerobic training—useful as well for warm-up and cool-down while lifting. If you already own a bicycle, you might select a wind trainer to turn your bike into a stationary bike, as we discussed in chapter 1. If you prefer a true exercise bike, there are many top-quality models to choose from (in the $250 to $500 price range). Or if you'd like the most complete aerobic workout possible, you could opt for a rowing machine. Some manufacturers have "souped up" their bikes and rowers with computers that time your workout, show cadence and tell you how many calories you are burning.

Depending on your budget and your affinity for expensive features, you can assemble a complete gym for under $200, over $2,000, or somewhere in between. Once you know what you're looking for, you are ready to begin shopping.

Shopping Tips

You walk into a store and there, on the "road to fitness," are countless exercise bikes, a dozen rowing machines, a few treadmills, cross-country ski simulators, rebounding trampolines and a gleaming array of multigyms and free weights. You scratch your head and wonder how you will ever make a choice. But not to worry—a little homework will help you make the right selection.

Before you spend any money, decide where you are going to use the equipment, and sketch out a floor plan for your gym. Consider how much floor space you have available and how much space is needed to comfortably use each machine.

As you are looking at the equipment, you will notice that many machines are scaled-down versions of the ones you have been using at your health club. This is because many manufacturers offer a model for commercial use as well as a model for the consumer. Find out at your club which units stand up to heavy-duty use, and compare features with the home models.

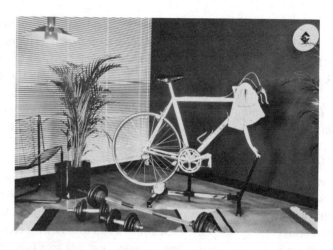

For under $200, you can mount your bike on a wind trainer ($90) and purchase a standard 110-pound set of free weights.

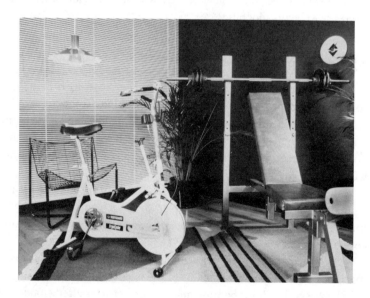

For under $750, you can select a high-quality exercise bike ($400) and a padded weight bench ($250) to increase the number of exercises you can safely perform with free weights.

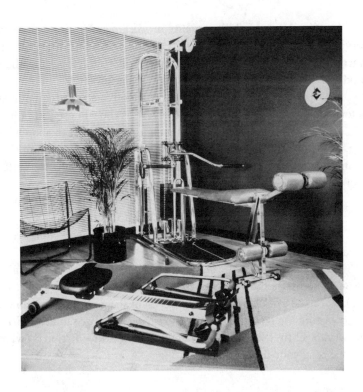

For over $2,000, you can construct the ultimate gym. A rowing machine ($600) provides an excellent full-body workout, and with a controlled-weight machine ($2,000 as shown), you can safely perform almost any exercise without a spotter.

When you are ready to talk to a salesperson, find one who can speak from experience. Ask the salesperson which particular equipment he or she has used and what the advantages and disadvantages are. A knowledgeable salesperson will answer your questions, help you assess your goals and match you with the equipment you will need.

Look into the safety features of each product. Is it safe to use alone? Are there any potential hazards, such as parts that may work loose or high-tension bands or springs that may cause injury?

Inquire about durability, quality of workmanship, warranty and service provided by the manufacturer or retailer. Read the fine print on warranty cards; reputable manufacturers will readily back up their products. Compare the product to other similar products.

Wear your workout clothes and shoes so you can try the equipment before you buy anything. Use the equipment as you will use it at home.

If others will be using the equipment, invite them to shop with you. Look for machines that will adjust quickly to keep your workout running smoothly. Nothing is as frustrating as having to stop after every set to prepare for the next exercise.

Check details on delivery and assembly. Unseen expenses here include shipping and handling charges and installation fees.

Shop around if you don't immediately find equipment to meet your needs and your budget.

Be cautious. Resist the temptation to buy machines that promise instant improvement. Items like spot-reducers and vibrating belts that claim to do the work for you are not overnight shape-making machines, and sweating the pounds away while wearing a rubber sauna suit isn't the way to get fit. (See the next chapter for more information on what *not* to spend your fitness dollars on.)

The Right Setup

Once the equipment is at home, be sure your "gym" is adequately ventilated and well lit. If you are an apartment dweller and you want your neighbors to keep talking to you, remember that a padded or carpeted floor will reduce noise. Mirrors are useful for checking form, and they create a nice illusion of "roominess."

After you have the essential equipment installed, your next goal is to make your home gym an enjoyable place. A television can relieve the monotony of cycling or rowing, and lively music on the stereo can be a terrific motivator. You can even invest in home exercise videos and records to add variety to your workouts.

And if you think you might miss the camaraderie found at a health club, you can simply invite your friends to your home gym for a workout and a postworkout meal—healthful food, of course, cooked just steps away in your very own kitchen.

More Equipment for Your Home Gym

If you're really serious about working out, you might want to consider a multistation gym to perform strength-training exercises. If you've started checking out the market, you'll know that there's a dizzying array of options, equipment and price tags to choose from.

This checklist should help you get started:

- Is the unit solidly constructed? If it is welded, are the welds clean and smooth? Cables, pulleys and all other parts of the lifting mechanism should be strong and operate smoothly. Keep your safety in mind.
- Is the machine easy to adjust for doing different exercises and using different amounts of weight?
- Are the benches and handgrips well padded, cushioned and durable enough to last?
- What are the unit's capabilities? Is there the right amount of weight to meet your needs? Can it be expanded or added to?
- Can you work out all the muscle groups you want to?
- Is the unit under warranty, and will the company stand by its product? Does the company have an authorized service agent or local representative to help you with problems?

Here are five multigym machines recommended by fitness experts we consulted:

The Lean Machine Pro.   This portable unit is one of the finest on the home market today, says Bob Goldman, D.O., chairman of the Amateur Athletic Union's Sports Medicine Committee. The machine is very compact and fits in a four- by six-foot space. Resistance can be adjusted in 1-pound increments from 30 to 200 pounds. The Lean Machine Pro uses a patented cam spring instead of weights to provide resistance. Cost: about $695. For more information, contact Inertia Dynamics Corporation, 7245 South Harl Avenue, Tempe, AZ 85283 (800-821-7143).

The Total Gym.   This is a well-made portable machine that uses your own weight for resistance. You lie on a glideboard and pull yourself up an incline using a pulley system. You can choose from 11 different resistance levels. Cost: about $595. Contact the West Bend Company, West Bend, WI 53095 (414-334-6909).

The Precor 720 Incline Exerciser.   This portable unit operates like The Total Gym, with 20 different incline settings to change the resistance. You can also alter the pulleys to change resistance. Cost: about $500. Contact Precor, P.O. Box 1018, Redmond, WA 98052 (800-662-0606).

Universal gym equipment.   Any multigym unit made by Universal is well worth its price, says Dr. Goldman. If you've ever worked out at a club or gym, you've surely seen the company's institutional units. The home versions are made with the same care and attention to design, detail and components. Universal's equipment provides resistance using weight stacks. The company makes three freestanding units for the home market, from a smaller machine (the Power-Pak 275) to two larger and more versatile units (the Power-Pak 300 and the Power-Pak 400). They range in price from $1,479 to $2,724, with optional equipment costing more. Contact Universal Fitness Products, P.O. Box 1270, Cedar Rapids, IA 52406 (800-553-7901).

Paramount fitness equipment.   Like Universal, any Paramount gym is worth its weight in gold, says Dr. Goldman. It also uses weight stacks for resistance. The company makes three units for the home market, from its smaller version (called the Fitness Mate) to two larger and more versatile units (the Fitness Trainer and the Fitness Trainer II). Basic prices range from $1,425 to $3,825, with optional equipment costing more. Contact Paramount Fitness Corporation, 6450 East Bandini Boulevard, Los Angeles, CA 90040 (800-421-6242).

Treadmills: Running When There's No Place to Go

Icy streets and early darkness may be keeping you from your outdoor running program. But a treadmill can put you back in action again, even if the scenery is a little monotonous. Tread in front of a television, however, and you've got a productive way to watch the evening news, a ball game or a video movie.

Treadmills come in two versions: motorized and nonmotorized. Your decision will likely be based on how much you want to spend—the motorized kind are pricier. But the two kinds have other pros and cons you may want to consider.

The nonmotorized treadmill operates using your own horsepower. The motorized type runs when you flick it on—but don't think you're getting less of a workout. The motor isn't making the exercise any easier for you; it's just carrying the running surface in the opposite direction from the one in which you're headed. One advantage of the nonmotorized treadmill is that it usually won't break down. A motorized treadmill could, and then you're out of commission until it's fixed.

But motorized treadmills have advantages if you have the money. First, they help you maintain a steady pace, thereby controlling your heart rate and giving you a better and more predictable workout. Second, since you're actually moving to keep up with the movement of the belt instead of propelling your body forward with each stride, the skeletal stress from heel-strike shock is minimized. That's good news if you're injury prone.

What should you look for if you're shopping for a treadmill? On motorized versions:

- Turn it on to find out if it has a quiet, heavy-duty motor.
- Make sure there's an easy-to-adjust variable speed control, so you can make your workouts harder or easier. The starting speed should be slow enough to allow walking; the high speed should be at least eight miles per hour.
- Look for an emergency on/off switch that's easy to reach.
- Front and/or side hand rails will help you keep your balance; a timer and odometer can quantify your workout.
- Many treadmills have an incline adjustment so you can simulate hill running for a more challenging workout.

On nonmotorized versions:

- Check to see that the rollers that cause the belt to move operate freely and without friction. Ask the dealer about how to keep them lubricated.
- Make sure the belt surface is comfortable and well padded.

- Try it out to find out if you get a smooth, quiet ride.
- Look for a timer, an odometer and front or side rails for balancing.

Here are a few models we've examined:

Precor treadmills.   While these machines all boast a 1-mile-per-hour minimum speed (slow enough for even elderly people), their top speeds range from 8 miles per hour (the model 910ei) and 10 miles per hour (the model 935e) to 12 miles per hour (the M series 9.5). All three are motorized. The 910ei and the M series 9.5 both have incline adjustment features. The 935e calculates your calorie expenditure. Prices range from $2,300 to $4,200. For more information, contact Precor, P.O. Box 1018, Redmond, WA 98052 (800-662-0606).

The Tredex 2924 and 2902.   For the home market, there are both a motorized and a nonmotorized treadmill. The Tredex 2924 is motorized, with speeds up to eight miles per hour. A computerized digital control panel shows you your speed, running time, distance and pace per mile. Cost: $2,895. The Tredex 2902 is Universal's nonmotorized model. It costs $1,246. For more information, contact Universal Fitness Products, P.O. Box 1270, Cedar Rapids, IA 52406 (800-553-7901).

The West Bend 8100.   The 8100 is a nonmotorized treadmill with a lot of the same features usually found on motorized versions. An electronic console gives your elapsed time, distance, running speeds and total accumulated miles. There's an incline adjustment and a fingertip adjustment knob to change the level of resistance. Cost: $649.95. For more information, contact the West Bend Company, P.O. Box 278, West Bend, WI 53095 (414-334-6909).

Gimmicks and Gadgets That Don't Work

There are countless manufacturers out there who want to slim your bulging belly by thinning out your wallet. From the novice to the pro, those wanting to lift weights and work out have almost as many gadgets to choose from as ice cream lovers have flavors. But when it comes to those shiny metal and leather gizmos, not all that glitters is fitness gold.

Dipping Belts

A dipping belt is a device used mostly by those well-conditioned folks who can—and want to—work their muscles overtime. For most of us, however, a workout without the added weight is sufficient to develop upper body strength.

Figure Trimmers

A figure trimmer may be a great device for doing the twist, but you'll never be able to call it exercise. For one thing, it's not demanding enough to work the muscles properly. The best way to "twist" the body into shape is with your own power.

Gravity Inversion Devices

People are going head over heels for gravity boots, which are used for hanging upside down to stretch back muscles and relieve the stress on joints. But researchers at the Chicago College of Osteopathic Medicine say that hanging upside down may be dangerous for some people, namely the elderly, those with glaucoma and those with high blood pressure. The position, the researchers say, raises blood pressure and pulse rate and puts extra pressure on the arteries of the eye, which can be dangerous for glaucoma patients.

Sauna Belts

A sauna belt may seem to whittle inches from your waistline, but what you're losing is water, not fat. The loss is only momentary. All that weight will come right back as soon as fluids are replenished. Cutting calories and exercising are the only ways to tighten the belt permanently.

Body Wraps

Want to lose a few fast pounds in a few short hours? Or whittle away inches with no effort at all?

That sounds too good to be true—and it is. Advertisements for body wraps claim all you need to do is lather your body with some "special" cream and wrap yourself up in cellophane (or other nonporous material) and presto—in less than an hour you're slimmer and trimmer. And it's true: In less than an hour you are slimmer and trimmer— but only for about another hour or so. After a few glasses of water your weight will be right back where it started. Because it's only water, *not* fat, that you shed in the body wrap.

As for the inches, well, they'll bounce back, too. If you twist a rubber band around your finger, leave it there and remove it a few minutes later, you'll have an indentation on your finger—a temporary one. The same thing happens if you wrap your body tightly in something—

whether it be cellophane or a girdle. The inches aren't lost, merely shifted. They'll creep back to normal in a matter of time.

So the answer's no. You're not bound for weight loss in a body wrap. Only disappointment.

Slant Boards

A slant board is a convenient and comfortable way to increase resistance and tighten the stomach muscles when doing Sit-Ups. But you should skip the added expense and the strain it puts on your lower back. You can get the same results by padding the floor and doing Sit-Ups with your knees bent and your feet flat.

Vibrating Machines

Is it really possible to shake, rattle or roll away fat? That's the claim made for those vibrating belt machines popular at some fitness centers. The idea is that you lean your tush against a wide belt that's hooked up to a jiggling machine. Your bottom wiggles—but will the fat wander? No way. An editorial in the *Journal of the American Medical Association* referred to a study on belt vibrators that proved they're ineffective. Not

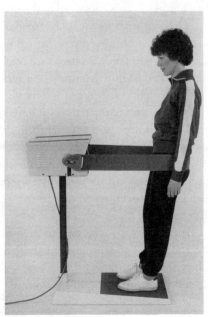

Vibrating Belt

only were they useless in reducing the thigh and hip area, but they didn't help with weight loss, either. You'd have to go through 307 15-minute sessions to use enough calories to burn one pound!

Bust Developers

About the only thing a bust developer builds up is the hopes of the person buying it. Unfortunately, the bust developer will never live up to its promise. A women's sports research expert states unequivocally that bust developer exercises do not increase mammary tissue. Likewise, a study at the University of Arizona of 34 women who underwent a 21-day development program found absolutely no benefits.

Can You Get Fit while You Sit?

As a folding chair it doesn't do badly, but as far as giving "an excellent aerobic and muscle-toning workout using all the large muscle groups at once," the Exerchair would do well to take a few giant steps backward to the drawing board.

"On a scale of one to ten, I'd have to give it about a two," said one certified fitness instructor who was asked to put the chair through its paces. "The device could be effective for toning individual muscle groups, but I found myself tiring out before getting into any sort of aerobic rhythm I could sustain."

Other testers of the Exerchair agreed. Four out of five complained of neck pain or other forms of discomfort that cut their workouts short of being aerobic. Testers complained, too, of the chair's inadequate brochure: Barely enough information is presented to acquaint users with the chair's basic workings, much less instruct them in movements capable of toning the entire body.

"As a device for achieving muscle tone in the areas of the back, shoulders and arms in people with compromised abilities— such as older folks or people unable to walk—the chair might hold some potential. But for the average person looking for a

Head Straps

Made of canvas, the head strap is a small harness and chain designed to hold barbell plates. It also can be attached to a pulley. Its purpose is to strengthen and develop the neck. To get the maximum benefits, be sure to get proper instructions before you attach the barbells or pulley and charge ahead. It's not a device recommended for the novice.

Exercise Wheels

Exercise wheels are advertised as an easy way to trim the midriff. While they do put stress on the stomach muscles when rolled back and

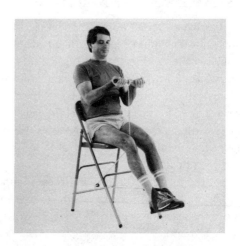

Exerchair

good aerobic workout in a hurry, the unit leaves a lot to be desired," the fitness instructor said. "A person would be better off with a rowing machine."

Nor is the Exerchair a bargain. The unit sells for $79.95 and is available from Exerchair, 10344 Dempster, Cupertino, CA 95014 (408-255-2588).

forth on the floor, they hardly get at the "gut" of the problem. In other words, they do nothing to rid the body of fat. Tightening stomach muscles is one way to fight the battle of the bulge, but ultimately, only exercise and diet work directly on body fat. This device may have appeal as a quick, fun way to slim down, but it may be just a way of putting off the real work of losing weight.

Weighted Belts

Putting on a ten-pound belt to jog or exercise is a minimally effective way to work the body harder. The same effect can be obtained by running up an incline, and you won't need to spend a dime. The principle's the same as working the body against gravity. Our advice: Don't buy it.

Passive Exercise Machines

"Passive exercise" won't help you get fit. You get only minimal results—for maximum expense. Being advertised for passive exercise is a device called an Electronic Muscle Stimulator (EMS). "It is nothing new," says Joyce Campbell, assistant professor of physical therapy at the University of Southern California. "Electrical stimulation devices have been used for years by physical therapists to treat trauma patients who have lost nerve supply to the muscles and patients recovering from long-term limb immobilization, strokes or spinal injury, and to relieve isolated joint pain."

But the role they can play in fitness is another story.

The way an EMS works is simple. You merely lie back and get wired to the machine's electrical currents. Most people report feeling a tingling sensation.

What happens, explains Campbell, is that electrical stimulation causes the muscles alternately to contract and relax. "There has been no documentation that EMS will help the normal person lose weight, increase stamina or build strength as effectively as voluntary exercise," she says. "And it is a not substitute for a regular exercise program, such as swimming or bicycling, in improving aerobic capacity.

"EMS is potentially dangerous and should not be used by those with electronic pacemakers or with cardiac arrhythmia," warns Campbell.